WORKBOOK

Counseling and Mental Health Services

Reno A. Palombit
Director of CTE for Johnston County Public Schools
Raleigh, North Carolina

Alyson L. McIntyre-Reiger, CFCS
Indiana FCCLA State Adviser
Executive Director for LEADFCS Education
Fountaintown, Indiana

Publisher
The Goodheart-Willcox Company, Inc.
Tinley Park, IL
www.g-w.com

ISBN 979-8-89118-923-2

1 2 3 4 5 6 7 8 9 – 26 – 29 28 27 26 25 24

The Goodheart-Willcox Company, Inc. Brand Disclaimer: Brand names, company names, and illustrations for products and services included in this text are provided for educational purposes only and do not represent or imply endorsement or recommendation by the author or the publisher.

The Goodheart-Willcox Company, Inc. Safety Notice: The reader is expressly advised to carefully read, understand, and apply all safety precautions and warnings described in this book or that might also be indicated in undertaking the activities and exercises described herein to minimize risk of personal injury or injury to others. Common sense and good judgment should also be exercised and applied to help avoid all potential hazards. The reader should always refer to the appropriate manufacturer's technical information, directions, and recommendations; then proceed with care to follow specific equipment operating instructions. The reader should understand these notices and cautions are not exhaustive.

The publisher makes no warranty or representation whatsoever, either expressed or implied, including but not limited to equipment, procedures, and applications described or referred to herein, their quality, performance, merchantability, or fitness for a particular purpose. The publisher assumes no responsibility for any changes, errors, or omissions in this book. The publisher specifically disclaims any liability whatsoever, including any direct, indirect, incidental, consequential, special, or exemplary damages resulting, in whole or in part, from the reader's use or reliance upon the information, instructions, procedures, warnings, cautions, applications, or other matter contained in this book. The publisher assumes no responsibility for the activities of the reader.

The Goodheart-Willcox Company, Inc. Internet Disclaimer: The Internet resources and listings in this Goodheart-Willcox Publisher product are provided solely as a convenience to you. These resources and listings were reviewed at the time of publication to provide you with accurate, safe, and appropriate information. Goodheart-Willcox Publisher has no control over the referenced websites and, due to the dynamic nature of the Internet, is not responsible or liable for the content, products, or performance of links to other websites or resources. Goodheart-Willcox Publisher makes no representation, either expressed or implied, regarding the content of these websites, and such references do not constitute an endorsement or recommendation of the information or content presented. It is your responsibility to take all protective measures to guard against inappropriate content, viruses, or other destructive elements.

Front Cover Image Credit. SDI Productions/E+ via Getty Images

Contents

Chapter 1 Introduction to Counseling and Mental Health 1
Lesson 1.1 Activity A Deinstitutionalization Debate 1
Lesson 1.1 Activity B Key Terms Review 3
Lesson 1.2 Activity C Key Terms Review 4
Lesson 1.2 Activity D Comparing Careers 5
Lesson 1.2 Activity E Specialties within Counseling and Social Work 6
Lesson 1.3 Activity F Key Terms Review 7
Lesson 1.3 Activity G Counselor Dispositions 8
Chapter 1 Activity H Chapter Review 9

Chapter 2 Relating to Self and Others 11
Lesson 2.1 Activity A Key Terms Review 11
Lesson 2.2 Activity B Exploring Your Emotions 12
Lesson 2.1 Activity C Bronfenbrenner's Ecological Systems Theory 13
Lesson 2.2 Activity D Key Terms Review 14
Lesson 2.2 Activity E Values Clarification 15
Lesson 2.2 Activity F Personality Assessments 17
Lesson 2.3 Activity G Key Terms Review 18
Lesson 2.3 Activity H Setting Boundaries 19
Lesson 2.3 Activity I Groups and Teams 20
Chapter 2 Activity J Chapter Review 21

Chapter 3 Relationships 23
Lesson 3.1 Activity A Attachment Theory 23
Lesson 3.1 Activity B Key Terms Review 24
Lesson 3.2 Activity C Key Terms Review 25
Lesson 3.2 Activity D Family Communication Styles 26
Lesson 3.3 Activity E Key Terms Review 27
Lesson 3.3 Activity F Setting Boundaries 28
Chapter 3 Activity G Chapter Review 29

Chapter 4 Mental Health Throughout the Life Span 31
Lesson 4.1 Activity A Key Terms Review 31
Lesson 4.1 Activity B Compare Developmental Theories 32
Lesson 4.2 Activity C Key Terms Review 33
Lesson 4.2 Activity D Protective Factors versus Risk Factors for ACEs 34
Lesson 4.2 Activity E Reading Charts – Mental Health Treatment for Children 35
Lesson 4.3 Activity F Key Terms Review 36
Lesson 4.3 Activity G Mental Health in Older Adulthood 37
Chapter 4 Activity H Chapter Review 39

Chapter 5 Communities and Mental Health....41
Lesson 5.1 Activity A Cultural Conversations....41
Lesson 5.1 Activity B Key Terms Review....43
Lesson 5.2 Activity C Key Terms Review....45
Lesson 5.2 Activity D Community Resource Mapping....46
Lesson 5.3 Activity E Volunteerism Statistics....47
Lesson 5.3 Activity F Key Terms Review....49
Lesson 5.3 Activity G Moral Development....50
Chapter 5 Activity H Chapter Review....51

Chapter 6 The Biology of Psychology....55
Lesson 6.1 Activity A Key Terms Review....55
Lesson 6.1 Activity B The Nervous System....56
Lesson 6.1 Activity C Neurotransmitter Research....57
Lesson 6.2 Activity D Key Terms Review....58
Lesson 6.2 Activity E Structure and Function....59
Lesson 6.3 Activity F Key Terms Review....61
Lesson 6.3 Activity G Sensation and Perception Scenarios....62
Chapter 6 Activity H Chapter Review....63

Chapter 7 Language and Learning....65
Lesson 7.1 Activity A Key Terms Review....65
Lesson 7.1 Activity B Promoting Early Language Learning....66
Lesson 7.2 Activity C Key Terms Review....67
Lesson 7.2 Activity D Memory Process Graphic Organizer....68
Lesson 7.3 Activity E Key Terms Review....69
Lesson 7.3 Activity F Divergent Thinking Exercise....70
Lesson 7.3 Activity G Gardner's Theory of Multiple Intelligences....71
Chapter 7 Activity H Chapter Review....72

Chapter 8 Neurodivergence....75
Lesson 8.1 Activity A Special Educator Interview....75
Lesson 8.1 Activity B Key Terms Review....77
Lesson 8.2 Activity C Key Terms Review....78
Lesson 8.2 Activity D The Watchman Theory....79
Lesson 8.3 Activity E Key Terms Review....81
Lesson 8.3 Activity F Reading and Understanding Data....82
Chapter 8 Activity G Chapter Review....84

Chapter 9 Mental Disorder....87
Lesson 9.1 Activity A Rosenhan's Pseudopatients....87
Lesson 9.1 Activity B Key Terms Review....89
Lesson 9.2 Activity C Key Terms Review....90
Lesson 9.2 Activity D Recognizing Symptoms....91
Lesson 9.2 Activity E Statistics of Disorders....93

Lesson 9.3 Activity F Key Terms Review....95
Lesson 9.3 Activity G Disorder Jeopardy....97
Chapter 9 Activity H Chapter Review....99

Chapter 10 Treatment....101
Lesson 10.1 Activity A Cognitive Distortions....101
Lesson 10.1 Activity B Key Terms Review....102
Lesson 10.2 Activity C Key Terms Review....103
Lesson 10.2 Activity D Recognizing Modalities....104
Lesson 10.2 Activity E Psychotropic Medication Research....105
Lesson 10.2 Activity F Treatment Data....107
Lesson 10.3 Activity G Key Terms Review....109
Lesson 10.3 Activity H Reflecting on a Specialty....110
Chapter 10 Activity I Chapter Review....111

Chapter 11 Navigating Life's Challenges....113
Lesson 11.1 Activity A Understanding Trauma....113
Lesson 11.1 Activity B Bullying Statistics....115
Lesson 11.1 Activity C Key Terms Review....117
Lesson 11.2 Activity D Key Terms Review....118
Lesson 11.2 Activity E Types of Grief and Grieving....119
Lesson 11.3 Activity F Key Terms Review....120
Lesson 11.3 Activity G Make the Connection....121
Chapter 11 Activity H Chapter Review....123

Chapter 12 Living with Integrity....127
Lesson 12.1 Activity A Key Terms Review....127
Lesson 12.1 Activity B Stages of Change Story....128
Lesson 12.2 Activity C Key Terms Review....129
Lesson 12.2 Activity D Personal Reflection....130
Lesson 12.2 Activity E Recognizing Empathy....131
Lesson 12.3 Activity F Key Terms Review....132
Lesson 12.3 Activity G Wellness Self-Assessment....133
Lesson 12.3 Activity H Practicing Gratitude....134
Chapter 12 Activity I Chapter Review....135

Chapter 13 School and Career Counseling....137
Lesson 13.1 Activity A Key Terms Review....137
Lesson 13.1 Activity B History of School Counseling Timeline....138
Lesson 13.2 Activity C Key Terms Review....139
Lesson 13.2 Activity D Student-to-School-Counselor Ratio....140
Lesson 13.2 Activity E School Counselor Informational Interview....141
Lesson 13.3 Activity F Key Terms Review....143
Lesson 13.3 Activity G Career Development Theories....144
Chapter 13 Activity H Chapter Review....147

Chapter 14 The Helping Relationship 149
Lesson 14.1 Activity A Key Terms Review 149
Lesson 14.1 Activity B Person-to-Person Relationship 150
Lesson 14.2 Activity C Key Terms Review 151
Lesson 14.2 Activity D Helping Skill Skits 152
Lesson 14.2 Activity E Practicing Helping Skills 153
Lesson 14.3 Activity F Key Terms Review 155
Lesson 14.3 Activity G Observing Counseling Sessions and Taking Notes 156
Lesson 14.3 Activity H Helper Self-Care 157
Chapter 14 Activity I Chapter Review 159

Chapter 15 The Business of Counseling and Mental Health 161
Lesson 15.1 Activity A Key Terms Review 161
Lesson 15.1 Activity B SWOT Analysis 162
Lesson 15.2 Activity C Patient Safety and Risk Management in Mental Health 163
Lesson 15.2 Activity D Key Terms Review 165
Lesson 15.3 Activity E Key Terms Review 166
Lesson 15.3 Activity F Entrepreneur Self-Assessment 167
Lesson 15.3 Activity G Exploring Nonprofit Organizations 168
Chapter 15 Activity H Chapter Review 169

Chapter 16 Your Career Development 171
Lesson 16.1 Activity A Key Terms Review 171
Lesson 16.1 Activity B Professional Association Recruitment Campaign 172
Lesson 16.1 Activity C Peer Mediation Activity 173
Lesson 16.1 Activity D Informational Interview 175
Lesson 16.1 Activity E Job Shadowing 176
Lesson 16.1 Activity F FCCLA Planning Process Activity 177
Lesson 16.2 Activity G Key Terms Review 178
Lesson 16.2 Activity H Practice Writing BAQQR Bullet Statements 179
Lesson 16.2 Activity I Job and Career Fair Preparation 180
Chapter 16 Activity J Chapter Review 181

Name ______________________ Date ____________ Class ____________

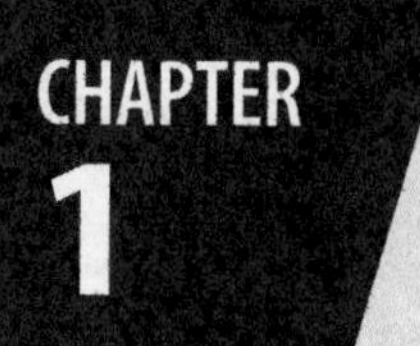

Introduction to Counseling and Mental Health

Lesson 1.1 Activity A

Deinstitutionalization Debate

Your class will be divided into two groups. You will either be For Deinstitutionalization (community-based mental healthcare) or Against Deinstitutionalization.

Part 1

Start by researching the arguments for and against deinstitutionalization or community-based mental healthcare. Be sure to cite sources and to use high-quality information. Summarize your key points/arguments below.

My Position (For or Against Deinstitutionalization)

____

Five Key Points For My Position

Key Point	Source

Three Key Points Against My Opponent's Position

Key Point	Source

(Continued)

Part 2

Working with a partner who has the same position as you, compare key points, arguments, and notes. Prepare for the debate by discussing the following with your partner:

- Do you think our key points are strong? How could they be stronger?
- How do you think they will challenge our key points and arguments? How could we respond to those challenges?
- How reputable or credible are our sources?

Make any changes to your key points above and take notes on another page that you can use during the debate. Then, participate in the debate as structured by your teacher.

Part 3

After the debate, reflect on your experience by answering the following debrief questions.

1. How did this activity affect your personal opinions or beliefs on this topic? Did they change them, reinforce them, and/or allow you to gain new insights into the complexity of the topic? Explain.

2. How did you think you performed in the debate? Was the experience difficult? What made it difficult?

3. What did you do well in the debate? What might you do differently in a future debate about a different topic?

Name ______________________ Date ______________ Class ____________

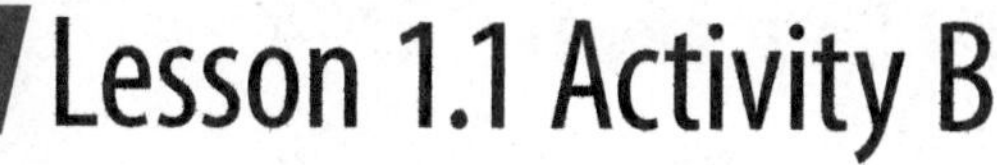

Lesson 1.1 Activity B

Key Terms Review

Part 1

Match the term with the correct example of the type of health.

1. _____ Coping with normal stresses of life
2. _____ Being self-aware of emotions
3. _____ Functioning of the body
4. _____ Working productively and contributing to community
5. _____ Forming meaningful relationships with others
6. _____ Coping with both positive and negative emotions
7. _____ Adapting comfortably in social situations

A. mental health
B. emotional health
C. social health
D. physical health

Part 2

Fill in the blanks in the following statements to review the lesson's key terms.

1. Historically, many women were diagnosed with a condition called _____, which was used to describe a set of symptoms such as anxiety, shortness of breath, nervousness, insomnia, or other related symptoms.

   ____

2. Using stone tools to chip a hole in the skull to release evil spirits believed to plague an individual is called _____.

   ____

3. The ability to function positively and feel a sense of satisfaction with one's life is called _____.

   ____

4. _____ is the absence of disease and a state of complete mental, social, and physical well-being.

   ____

5. A hero may make amends, or _____, for their failures.

   ____

6. The _____ _____ movement describes the shift away from institutionalized care in asylums toward outpatient care oriented around the community.

   ____

7. The _____ _____ mental healthcare model relies on a range of treatment options including community mental health centers and small residential homes.

   ____

8. Forming an organized whole that functions effectively with little effort through the process of bringing together a person's traits, behavior patterns, and motives is called _____ _____ _____.

   ____

Name ______________________ Date ____________ Class ____________

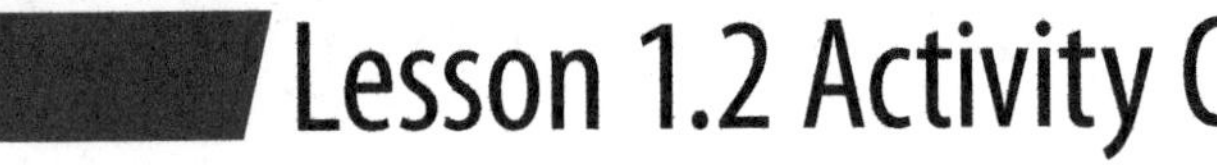

Lesson 1.2 Activity C

Key Terms Review

Part 1

Review the lesson's key terms by matching the term with the example.

1. _____ A self-employed mental health professional setting
2. _____ Scientific study of the mind and behavior
3. _____ A field that promotes social change and empowerment of people and communities
4. _____ A branch of medicine focused on the diagnosis and treatment of mental illness, emotional disturbance, and abnormal behavior
5. _____ The environment where counselors and mental health professionals work and the nature of their work
6. _____ A field in which practitioners assist and guide people to resolve problems or difficulties
7. _____ A set of abilities used to form relationships and communicate with other people
8. _____ A practitioner that typically treats patients through psychotherapy
9. _____ The concepts, terms, and activities that make up a professional field

A. body of knowledge
B. clinical psychologist
C. counseling
D. interpersonal skills
E. practice setting
F. private practice
G. psychiatry
H. psychology
I. social work

Part 2

Answer the following question.

1. List three types of professional counselors.

____

____

____

____

Name ______________________ Date ____________ Class ____________

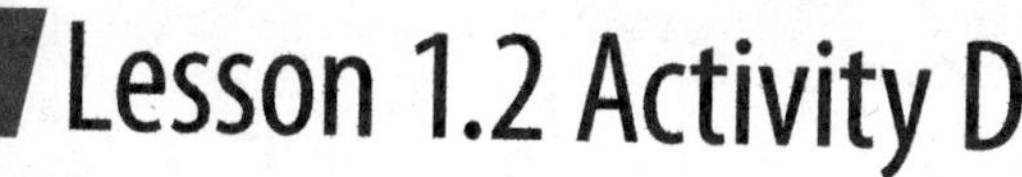

Lesson 1.2 Activity D

Comparing Careers

Read each statement and select the career that is least likely *to relate to that statement. If you are unsure, research the career online to learn more about their work.*

1. _____ Works one-on-one with clients providing licensed counseling services
   A. Clinical psychologist
   B. Life coach
   C. Clinical social worker
2. _____ Prescribes medications that treat mental health conditions
   A. Clinical psychologist
   B. Psychiatrist
   C. Psychiatric nurse practitioner
3. _____ Uses psychotherapy to treat clients in a clinical practice setting
   A. Mental health counselor
   B. Research psychologist
   C. Behavioral health therapist
4. _____ Uses social psychology to resolve conflict between employees or apply educational psychology to develop lessons and training programs
   A. Clinical psychologist
   B. Human resources manager
   C. Teacher
5. _____ Monitors vital signs and helps people participate in therapeutic and recreational activities
   A. Mental and behavioral health technician
   B. Psychiatric registered nurse
   C. Hospital social worker
6. _____ Develops and implements mental health interventions among groups, teams, or geographic areas, rather than individuals
   A. Community social worker
   B. Industrial-organizational psychologist
   C. Marriage and family therapist
7. _____ Works with students to help remove barriers to learning
   A. Career counselor
   B. School counselor
   C. School social worker
8. _____ Helps people navigate challenges in their professional life and roles at work
   A. Mental health counselor
   B. School social worker
   C. Career counselor
9. _____ Helps people overcome disorders related to substance use
   A. Bereavement counselor
   B. Substance use counselor
   C. Behavioral health social worker
10. _____ Advocates for the rights and protection of children, older adults, and marginalized communities
    A. Social worker
    B. Social psychologist
    C. Forensic psychologist

Name ______________________ Date ____________ Class ____________

Lesson 1.2 Activity E

Specialties within Counseling and Social Work

In your textbook, Figure 1.9 describes types of professional counselors and Figure 1.10 describes specialties in social work. Select and research one occupation from each area, utilizing the Occupational Outlook Handbook *and other job sources. Complete the following outline, and then answer the reflection question.*

Counseling Specialty

1. Name of occupation:

____

2. Brief description of the specialization:

____

____

Job Information Categories	Responses from Research
Median Pay	
Entry Level Education	
Work Experience in a Related Occupation	
On-the-Job Training	
Job Outlook	

Social Work Specialty

1. Name of occupation:

____

2. Brief description of the specialization:

____

____

Job Information Categories	Responses from Research
Median Pay	
Entry Level Education	
Work Experience in a Related Occupation	
On-the-Job Training	
Job Outlook	

Reflection

1. Compare and contrast the two career specializations. Is there one that you are more interested in pursuing?

____

____

____

Name ______________________ Date ______________ Class ____________

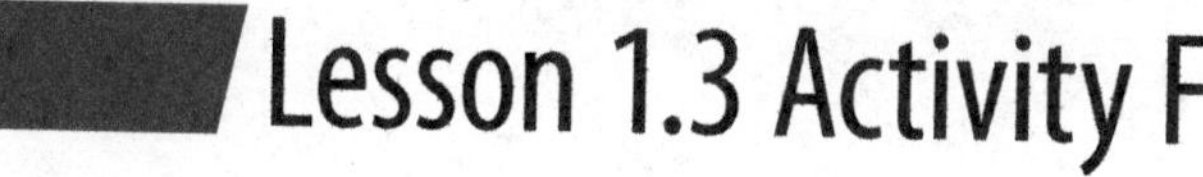

Lesson 1.3 Activity F

Key Terms Review

Part 1

Answer the following questions to review the lesson's key terms.

1. What are the beliefs and attitudes shared among colleagues in the counseling field that are grounded in the core values of the profession?

 ____

2. What is a place or environment in which a person can feel confident that they will not be exposed to discrimination, criticism, harassment, or any other emotional or physical harm?

 ____

3. What are skills specific to the work-related tasks of a job?

 ____

4. What are skills related to how an individual works and interacts with other people?

 ____

5. What is the experience of choosing to act rather than feeling pressured to act?

 ____

6. What are naturally recurring patterns of thought, feeling, or behavior that can be productively applied?

 ____

7. What are skills that allow individuals to analyze, reason, solve problems, plan, organize, and make sound decisions?

 ____

Part 2

Classify the following examples as a representation of critical-thinking, personal, or technical skills.

1. _____ Building rapport with individuals, families, and communities
2. _____ Using counseling treatment methods and techniques
3. _____ Being self-aware and emotionally stable during counseling sessions
4. _____ Questioning to better understand clients
5. _____ Using computer software to manage client records
6. _____ Applying project management skills to organize a project
7. _____ Problem-solving to help individuals overcome barriers to well-being
8. _____ Setting boundaries around work and personal life

A. Critical-thinking skills
B. Personal skills
C. Technical skills

Name ______________________________ Date ______________ Class ______________

Lesson 1.3 Activity G

Counselor Dispositions

For each scenario, describe how the counselor is exemplifying, or not exemplifying, one or more of the counselor dispositions.

Scenario A: Rashawn is working with a client. After their second session, Rashawn suspects the client is in an abusive relationship. He says, "You are in an abusive relationship. When you get home, I want you to pack a bag and move out."

____

____

____

____

Scenario B: Tabitha is working with a client who is resistant to therapy. The client uses many strategies to avoid a counseling relationship with her. Tabitha remains patient and continues to try different approaches to connect with her client.

____

____

____

____

Scenario C: Pluto is a counselor with strong religious beliefs. They work with a client who is anti-religious. The client is not showing any signs of having difficulty understanding their existence or making meaning of life. Without the client's input, Pluto develops a therapeutic goal to begin practicing a religion.

____

____

____

____

Scenario D: Quan's client shares that his partner called him out in front of their friends last week for saying something insensitive and judgmental. Quan asks, "How did that make you feel?" The client explains how small and ashamed he felt and how he wishes he was not so judgmental about people. Quan responds, "We all struggle with being too judgmental. But tell me more about what you said and why you think you said it."

____

____

____

____

Name ________________________ Date ____________ Class ____________

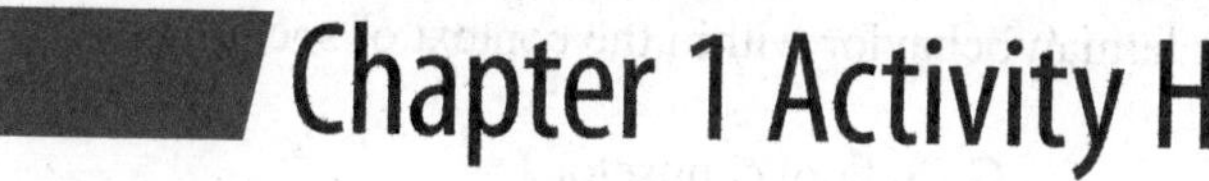

Chapter 1 Activity H

Chapter Review

Lesson 1.1 Perspectives on Counseling and Mental Health

Answer the following questions.

1. Tracey participates in a science book club. As part of the book club, they read nonfiction books about science and discuss and debate the content of the book. Which two dimensions of health and well-being does this activity support?

____

2. Andrew is seeking treatment for a substance use disorder. He is in the process of listening to and understanding how his behaviors have impacted the people in his life, acknowledging and owning his wrongdoings, and apologizing to them. This represents which phase in the hero's journey?

____

3. Name one historical mental health "illness" that is no longer categorized as a mental health condition today.

____

For each of the statements below, indicate True or False. If False, indicate how the statement would be changed to make it True.

4. Fear drove early humans' attempts to understand and treat mental health conditions.

____

5. English people were the first to attribute the brain as the source of mental function.

____

6. For the last 2,000 years, the theory of the four humors was the only one to describe the source of mental and emotional illness in Europe and the United States.

____

7. Dorothea Dix advocated for state-run asylums that promoted moral treatment of those with mental illness.

____

Lesson 1.2 The Counseling and Mental Health Career Pathway

Answer the following questions.

1. _____ In which practice setting does a mental health clinician work for themself?
   A. Government
   B. Hospital
   C. Private Practice
   D. School

2. _____ Which type of psychologist is *most likely* working with individual clients to heal mental health illness?
   A. Clinical psychologist
   B. Consumer psychologist
   C. Forensic psychologist
   D. Industrial-organizational psychologist

3. _____ Which counselor is *most likely* to help parents develop positive, healthy relationships with their children?
   A. Bereavement counselor
   B. Career counselor
   C. Marriage and family counselor
   D. Substance use counselor

(Continued)

4. _____ Which career pathway *most* involves understanding human behavior within the context of social, economic, and cultural systems?
   A. Psychiatrist
   B. Psychologist
   C. School counselor
   D. Social worker

5. _____ All of the following practitioners may be licensed to treat mental illness, *except* a _____.
   A. clinical social worker
   B. life coach
   C. mental health counselor
   D. psychiatric nurse practitioner

6. _____ Which career path is *least* related to counseling and mental health?
   A. Agriculture
   B. Healthcare
   C. Human resources
   D. Teaching and education

Lesson 1.3 Competence in Counseling and Mental Health

Answer the following questions.

1. The counselor regards others as capable of dealing with problems in their lives. They see people as worthy of _____ and _____.

   ____

2. The counselor is concerned with warm understanding and open-minded _____ of others and _____ of their viewpoints.

   ____

3. Strengths are developed by investing _____ and _____ into one's talent, knowledge, and skills.

   ____

4. _____ Applying techniques for notetaking, record keeping, and maintaining client confidentiality are all examples of _____.
   A. applied knowledge
   B. personal skills
   C. technical skills
   D. thinking skills

5. _____ Setting boundaries and being self-aware and emotionally stable are examples of _____.
   A. applied knowledge
   B. personal skills
   C. technical skills
   D. thinking skills

6. _____ Reading and writing literacy are examples of _____.
   A. applied knowledge
   B. personal skills
   C. technical skills
   D. thinking skills

7. _____ Asking the right questions and reading between the lines are examples of _____.
   A. applied knowledge
   B. personal skills
   C. technical skills
   D. thinking skills

For each statement below, indicate "T" for true or "F" for false as to whether it is a characteristic of brave and safe spaces.

8. _____ People make fun of others when they are outside of the space.
9. _____ Limits on confidentiality are clearly communicated.
10. _____ People stay curious and withhold judgment.
11. _____ People are reduced to their mistakes or accomplishments.
12. _____ People believe that everyone is trying their best.
13. _____ People are flawed and worthy of love and belonging in the space.

Name ________________________________ Date ________________ Class ____________

CHAPTER 2 Relating to Self and Others

Lesson 2.1 Activity A

Key Terms Review

Fill in the blanks in the following statements to review the lesson's key terms.

1. _____ is when a social worker recognizes that environmental context is important to understanding the individual.

   ____

2. _____ are the ways and means people use to meet their needs.

   ____

3. A(n) _____ is a group of interacting or interrelated elements that act according to a set of rules to form a unified whole.

   ____

4. _____ refers to an individual's perception about the underlying main causes of events in their life.

   ____

5. _____ places a higher value on the needs and goals of the individual, while _____ places a higher value on the needs and the goals of the group.

   ____

6. _____ is the realization of one's full potential.

   ____

7. A theory that argues that a person's environment affects every facet of their life, including their thoughts, feelings, and preferences is called _____.

   ____

8. The ability to understand one's emotions, to listen to others and empathize with their emotions, is called _____.

   ____

9. _____ is the study of how an individual's behaviors and environment can cause changes that affect the way genes work.

   ____

Name ______________________ Date ____________ Class __________

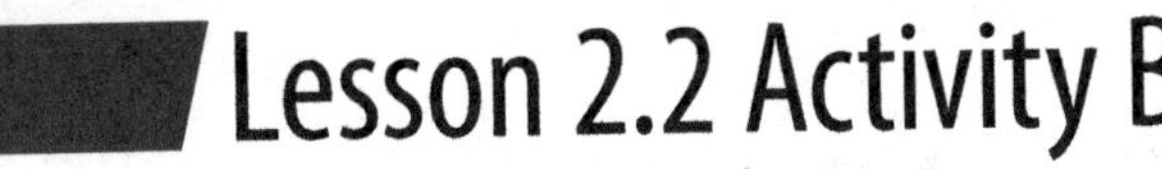

Lesson 2.2 Activity B

Exploring Your Emotions

Figure 2.2 provides a framework for exploring a person's emotions and responses to emotions. Reflect on a time you felt an emotion strongly. It can be a positive or negative emotion. Use that experience to complete the table below.

Reflection Questions	Response
Biology What sensations, feelings, or reactions occurred in your body? Did your body expand and take up more space or shrink and take up less space?	
Biography How did your family, community, and culture contribute to your experience? What messages validated or invalidated your emotions?	
Behavior What behaviors did you perform in reaction to the situation or emotion? Consider impulses and things you said and did. For example, did you get confrontational, want to be alone, or want to be with others?	
Backstory What relevant experiences, mindsets, or situational factors are important to understanding your experience? For example, what was your mood prior to the situation? What triggered the emotion?	

Name ______________________ Date ____________ Class ____________

Lesson 2.1 Activity C

Bronfenbrenner's Ecological Systems Theory

Part 1

Label the systems in Bronfenbrenner's Ecological Systems Theory. List the indicated number of examples for each system.

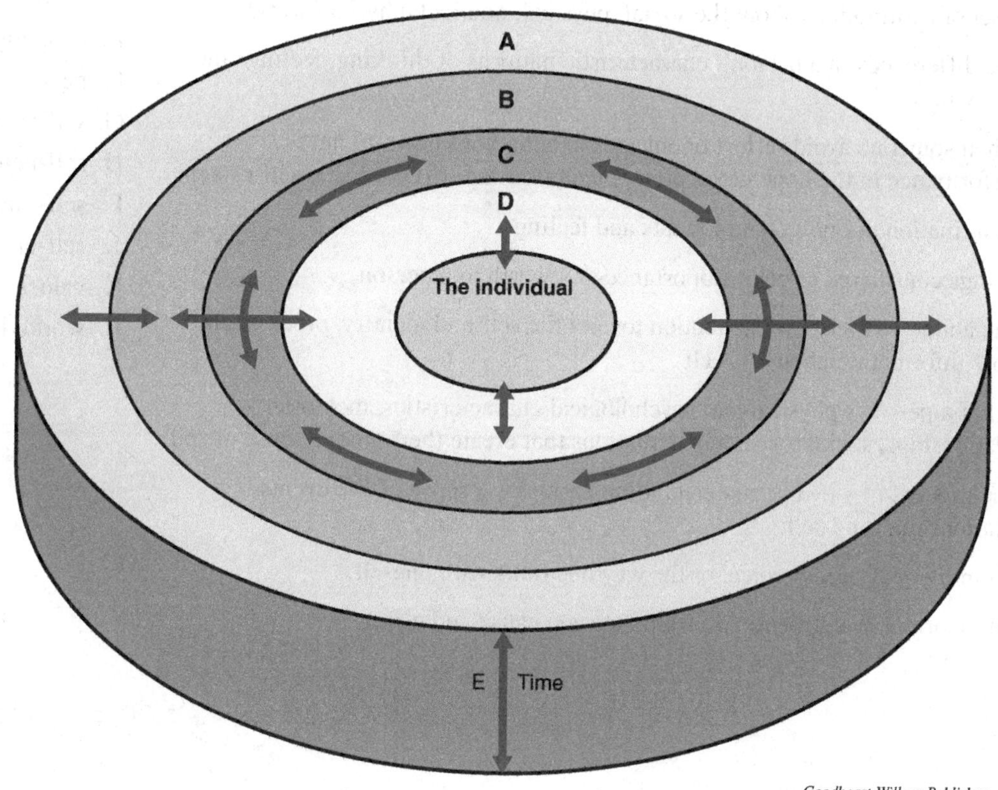

Goodheart-Willcox Publisher

Label	System	Examples
A		Three examples:
B		Two examples:
C		Three examples:
D		Two examples:
E		One example:

Name ______________________ Date ______________ Class ______________

Lesson 2.2 Activity D

Key Terms Review

Review the lesson's key terms by matching the term with the example.

1. _____ Things a person accepts as true, real, or valid
2. _____ A combination of the image you hold about yourself and your traits and the judgments you make about those traits
3. _____ A set of assumptions about the social, physical, and metaphysical world
4. _____ The differences in a person's characteristic patterns of thinking, feeling, and behaving
5. _____ When someone avoids effort or engages in behavior known to hurt performance in the hope of keeping potential failure from hurting self-esteem
6. _____ Examination of one's own thoughts and feelings
7. _____ Things considered to be of importance and worth to a person
8. _____ The ability to focus one's attention toward the self and identify, process, and store information about the self
9. _____ All of a person's physical and psychological characteristics, memories, relationships, social roles, and affiliations that create their unique sense of self
10. _____ The process of viewing, understanding, or making sense of life events, relationships, and self
11. _____ An individual's inner voice, or the way one talks with oneself
12. _____ An incorrect or untrue relationship between cause and effect

A. beliefs
B. causal fallacy
C. identity
D. introspection
E. meaning-making
F. personality
G. self-awareness
H. self-perception
I. self-sabotaging
J. self-talk
K. values
L. worldview

Name ______________________________ Date ______________ Class ____________

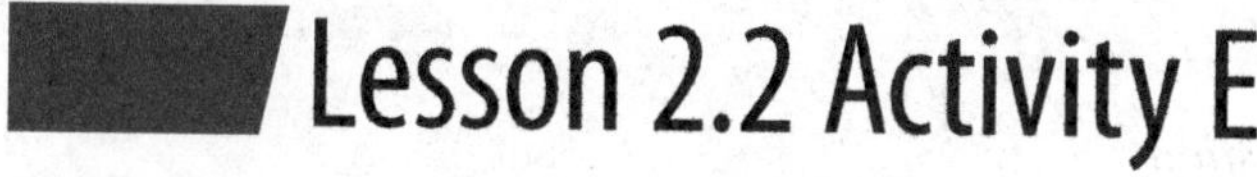

Lesson 2.2 Activity E

Values Clarification

Part 1

Place an "X" by your top 10 values.

	Accountability		Diversity		Home		Peace
	Adventure		Efficiency		Honesty		Playfulness
	Ambition		Empathy		Humor		Power
	Authenticity		Empowerment		Inclusion		Respect
	Beauty		Enthusiasm		Independence		Responsibility
	Belonging		Environment		Innovation		Selflessness
	Bravery		Ethical		Insightful		Self-reliance
	Career		Family		Intelligence		Sensitivity
	Charity		Financial stability		Justice		Service
	Community		Freedom		Kindness		Simplicity
	Compassion		Friendship		Love		Spirituality
	Competence		Fun		Loyalty		Success
	Cooperation		Generosity		Maturity		Thoughtfulness
	Courage		Grace		Optimism		Tradition
	Creativity		Gratitude		Order		Truth
	Curiosity		Growth		Originality		Toughness
	Decisiveness		Hard work		Passion		Uniqueness
	Dependability		Harmony		Patience		Wealth
	Discipline		Health		Patriotism		Wisdom

Of your top 10 values, identify and rank in order your top 5 core values. If you are having difficulty deciding, imagine a situation where you would have to choose one over another.

Ranking	Core Value
1	
2	
3	
4	
5	

(Continued)

Part 2

Reflecting on your top five values, answer the following questions.

1. In what ways do you live out your values? Consider how you spend your time and money and where you direct your attention.

____

____

____

____

____

____

2. How do you think clarifying one's values encourages authenticity, integration, and a sense of self?

____

____

____

____

____

____

3. Reflect on a time when a situation or person put you in a position that was in conflict with one of your values. What did that experience feel like?

____

____

____

____

____

4. In what ways do you think your family, community, or culture influenced your values?

____

____

____

____

____

5. How do you think your values may influence your future plans and goals?

____

____

____

Name ____________________ Date __________ Class __________

Lesson 2.2 Activity F

Personality Assessments

Take a personality assessment as directed by your teacher. Then, complete the reflection questions.

1. After reading your results, which parts of your results do you think are accurate or true about yourself?

2. Is there anything you disagree with or believe to be inaccurate? If yes, what?

3. What did you find interesting? What sparked curiosity about your self-perception?

4. How did the assessment help improve your self-awareness?

5. How might you use any insights gleaned from this assessment in the future?

Name ______________________ Date ____________ Class ____________

Lesson 2.3 Activity G

Key Terms Review

Answer the following questions to review the lesson's key terms.

1. What is a person's ability to understand the perspectives of other individuals, groups, or communities and to apply that understanding in interactions with them?

   ____

2. What is a measure of a person's social maturity and intelligence, or their ability to understand people and effectively relate to them?

   ____

3. What is the process of turning thoughts into a communicable message?

   ____

4. What is a measure of a person's emotional intelligence, including their ability to process emotional information and use it in reasoning and other cognitive activities?

   ____

5. What is the intervention of a neutral third person to help resolve a conflict?

   ____

6. What is the transmission of information, which may be by verbal or nonverbal means?

   ____

7. What is the ability to recognize, name, and understand one's feelings?

   ____

8. What is the ability to control one's response to emotions by anticipating outcomes?

   ____

9. What is a term that describes the process of interpreting a message?

   ____

10. What occurs when individuals change their language or style of language depending on the context?

    ____

11. What model characterizes the elements that feed drama?

    ____

12. What is the strength and extent of interpersonal connection existing among the members of a group?

    ____

Name ____________________ Date ____________ Class ____________

Lesson 2.3 Activity H

Setting Boundaries

Setting boundaries can help you keep healthy relationships or identify unhealthy relationships. Review Figure 2.16 to see examples of boundaries people may set in specific relationships. Review the following scenarios and describe a boundary you would set.

1. Scenario 1: You are working in a clinic and your shift ends at 4:30 p.m. You have many activities and responsibilities after work. Three days this week, your supervisor has asked to speak to you close to 4:30. On two of the days, you were still at work at 5:00 p.m.

   What boundary would you set?

   ____

   ____

   ____

   ____

   ____

   ____

2. Scenario 2: You are a 16-year-old living with your parents. Your parents require you to keep your phone downstairs at night when you go to bed. When you get up, you notice that your text messages were read and some even had responses sent. Your older sister says, "Yeah, I answered your texts for you this morning."

   What boundary would you set? What conversations might you have with your parents and sister?

   ____

   ____

   ____

   ____

   ____

   ____

3. Scenario 3: You tell your best friend a secret. The next day at school, you hear your friend sharing the secret with a group of classmates.

   What boundary would you set?

   ____

   ____

   ____

   ____

   ____

   ____

Name ____________________ Date __________ Class __________

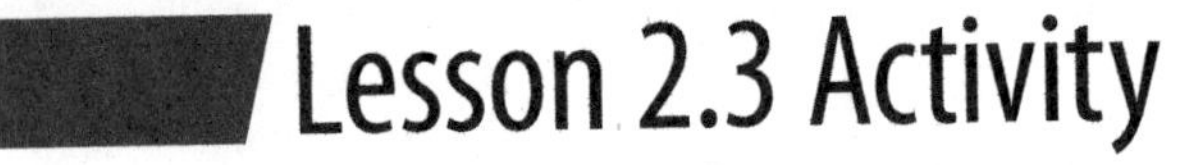

Lesson 2.3 Activity I

Groups and Teams

Imagine you are working with a team as an industrial-organizational psychologist. For each team dysfunction, suggest what the potential impact on the team may be and an intervention or strategy that could help improve the team's function.

Dysfunction	Indicator	Potential Impact	Intervention or Strategy
Absence of Trust	An unwillingness to be vulnerable; hiding or falsifying motives		
Fear of Conflict	Artificial harmony; lack of debate; guarded comments		
Lack of Commitment	Continual need for consensus and certainty; lack of buy-in to decisions; lots of second guessing		
Avoidance of Accountability	Unwillingness to call peers out on statements and behaviors; inability to separate personal from team relationship		
Inattention to Results	Individual (or home organization) needs take priority over collective team needs; goal is to exist (being on team is "enough")		

Name ______________________ Date ______________ Class ______________

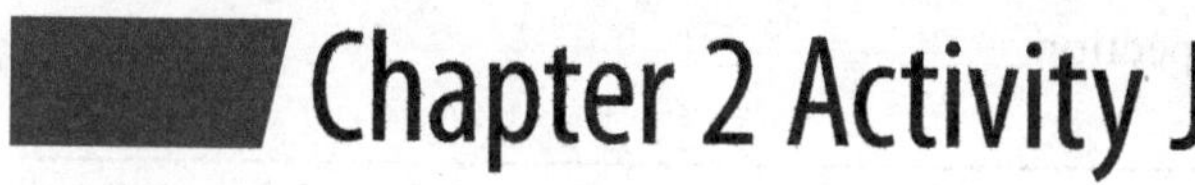

Chapter 2 Activity J

Chapter Review

Lesson 2.1 Understanding Human Systems

Answer the following questions.

1. _____ Which is *true* of human development?
   A. Mostly impacted by environmental factors
   B. Mostly impacted by genetic factors
   C. Impacted by environmental and genetic factors
   D. Neither impacted by environmental nor genetic factors
2. _____ Why is emotional literacy important?
   A. Understand one's own emotions.
   B. Empathize with others.
   C. Express emotions.
   D. All answers apply.
3. Explain a criticism of Maslow's Hierarchy of Needs.

____

____

Each of the following terms is an example of a fundamental human need from the Max-Neef Model of Human Scale Development. Match each term with the fundamental human need to which it best relates.

4. _____ Libraries
5. _____ Authenticity
6. _____ Parties
7. _____ Medicine
8. _____ Government
9. _____ Autonomy
10. _____ Art
11. _____ Career
12. _____ Hugs

A. subsistence
B. protection
C. affection
D. understanding
E. participation
F. leisure
G. creation
H. identity
I. freedom

For each statement below, indicate if it exemplifies an internal ("I") or external ("E") locus of control.

13. _____ "My passion and hard work have helped me achieve success."
14. _____ "Why bother trying? Whatever is meant to be will be."
15. _____ "Thanks! I was just lucky."
16. _____ "Luck is when preparation meets opportunity."
17. _____ "I set goals and create plans to achieve them."
18. _____ "I'll just wait and see what happens."

Lesson 2.2 Relationship with Self

Indicate whether each of the following statements is True or False. If False, correct the statement to make it True.

1. Personality encompasses all of a person's physical and psychological characteristics, memories, relationships, social roles, and affiliations that create their unique sense of self.

____

2. Personality is enduring and static.

____

(Continued)

3. Personality assessments can provide a foundation for introspection.

____

4. Introspection is the examination of one's own conscious thoughts and feelings.

____

Answer the following questions.

5. _____ Clarifying your values involves all of the following, *except* ______.
   A. inventory
   B. probing
   C. prioritizing
   D. self-improvement

6. _____ James believes his cancer diagnosis is teaching him how short and valuable his time on Earth is. This *best* exemplifies ______.
   A. meaning-making
   B. personality
   C. self-perception
   D. worldview

7. Self-perception is a combination of the image you hold about yourself and your traits (______) and the judgments you make about those traits (______).

____

8. _____ Latrice wants to be in a romantic relationship, but each time a person displays an interest in her, she criticizes or avoids them. This *best* exemplifies ______.
   A. self-esteem
   B. self-sabotaging
   C. self-awareness
   D. self-talk

Lesson 2.3 Interpersonal Relationships

Answer the following question.

1. _____ Which skill is *not* a part of one's emotional quotient (EQ)?
   A. Access and evoke emotions
   B. Recognize emotions accurately
   C. Regulate one's own and others' emotions to promote well-being
   D. Understand the perspectives of other individuals, groups, or communities

Match each example with the corresponding context for communication.

2. _____ Client-counselor
3. _____ Counselor's office
4. _____ Professional treatment
5. _____ Emotional distress
6. _____ Client's demographic profile

A. Physical context
B. Psychological context
C. Relational context
D. Social context
E. Cultural context

Answer the following question.

7. _____ Aliah, Robin, and Cornelius are co-workers in a drama triangle. Who is helping to dismantle the drama triangle?
   A. Robin feels Cornelius is a bully but that there is nothing she can do.
   B. Aliah's self-worth is tied to being helpful and making Robin feel better.
   C. Cornelius believes Robin is being too sensitive and needs to focus on meeting their quarterly goals.
   D. No one is helping to dismantle the drama triangle.

For each statement below, indicate the stage of group development: forming, storming, norming, or performing.

8. _____ Team members focus on the work, build relationships, and enjoy each other's company.
9. _____ Members get to know one another.
10. _____ People inside and outside the team can see the impact of the team's work.
11. _____ Teams encounter conflict.

Name ______________________ Date ____________ Class ____________

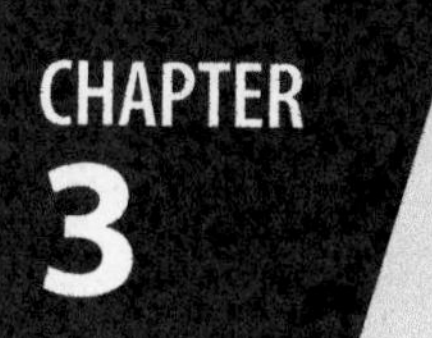

Relationships

Lesson 3.1 Activity A

Attachment Theory

For each principle of attachment theory, review the text and complete the reflection questions. You may need to use the internet to research principles more deeply.

Connection is a primary need.

Question	Response
What evidence is there that connection is a primary need of humans?	

Connection provides a safe haven.

Reflect on a time when you were in a stressful situation, and connection with another person helped you through it.

Question	Response
How did you feel before connecting with someone?	
How did you feel while connecting with someone?	
How did you feel after connecting with someone?	

Balance promotes a positive sense of self.

Question	Response
Describe how emotional balance promotes connection.	

Name ______________________________ Date ______________ Class ____________

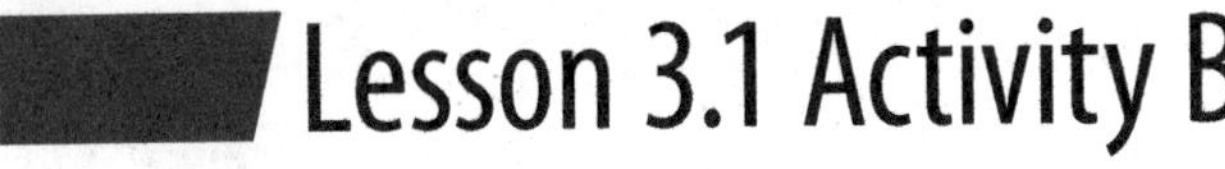

Lesson 3.1 Activity B

Key Terms Review

Part 1

Fill in the blanks in the following statements to review the lesson's key terms.

1. _____ suggests that the quality and characteristics of the bond formed between a child and their primary caregiver determines how the child will relate to others throughout their life.

   ____

2. An emotional disturbing experience or physical injury causing someone lasting shock is called _____.

   ____

3. The clinical term for overreacting is called _____.

   ____

4. A deep and enduring emotional bond between two people in which each seeks closeness is called _____.

   ____

5. _____ is abnormal alertness.

   ____

6. _____ occurs when an individual continuously faces a negative, uncontrollable situation and stops trying to change their circumstances.

   ____

7. A(n) _____ is an interdependent connection between people.

   ____

8. Emotional numbing and disconnection between body and feelings is called _____.

   ____

9. _____ occurs when a person chooses to turn toward another person to ask for help.

   ____

10. A group of conditions that result from experiencing an abnormal amount of stress in response to a stressful event is called _____.

    ____

Part 2

Choose the type of attachment based on the example given.

1. _____ Prone to fighting
2. _____ Demonstrates both anxious and avoidance behaviors
3. _____ Prone to fleeing
4. _____ Minimizes needs and shuts down
5. _____ Overly needy

A. Anxious Attachment
B. Avoidant Attachment
C. Fearful-Avoidant Attachment

Name ________________________ Date ____________ Class ________

Lesson 3.2 Activity C

Key Terms Review

Part 1

Review the lesson's key terms by matching the term with the example.

1. _____ To be counted on
2. _____ Groups of people who are related by genetics, marriage, or choice and who share resources
3. _____ Questions that assess the client's internal experience and help them work through parts of it
4. _____ Owning up to failures and shortcomings, both your own and others, and then working to repair the situation
5. _____ When someone can maintain their own thoughts and feelings despite the presence and pressure of close, intimate relationships
6. _____ The nervous unease that swirls within an interconnected group of people
7. _____ When you perform an action or behavior contrary to the emotions you feel
8. _____ When a person can distinguish between thoughts and feelings

A. accountable
B. families
C. incongruent behavior
D. interpersonal differentiation
E. intrapsychic differentiation
F. processing questions
G. reckoning
H. system anxiety

Part 2

Identify the Satir Family Communication style based on the incongruent behavior given.

1. Expresses a range of emotions and behaviors to avoid an issue.

____

2. Initiates conflict and projects toughness.

____

3. There are no incongruent behaviors.

____

4. Plays the role of peacemaker and peacekeeper.

____

5. Cold, unfeeling, and behaves the "correct" way.

____

Name ______________________________ Date ______________ Class ______________

Lesson 3.2 Activity D

Family Communication Styles

Read the story below and identify which family member exemplifies each of Satir's Family Communication Styles. Then, answer the final reflection question.

The Jones family is sitting around the dinner table enjoying their annual Thanksgiving meal when Elena blurts out, "Why are none of us saying what we are all thinking? This is ridiculous. Sam, none of us want to go to your house for Christmas!" The matriarch of the family, Diana, interjects, "Now is neither the time nor the place. We are having a nice family dinner. Now, who would like coffee with dessert?"

As Diana goes to start a pot of coffee, Mona starts to tear up, slams her silverware down, shouting angrily as she leaves the dining room. Rose quickly follows her outside and asks, "What's wrong, Mona?" Mona replies, "I'm so sick of how Elena talks to all of us! It makes me so angry, I can't handle it!" Rose responds, "I agree with you. That was uncalled for. But you know how she is, she's always been like that. Just breathe, let's calm down and we can head back in." They head back to the table. As they make their way back to their seats, Rose makes a face at Elena suggesting equal parts annoyance and hopeful relief. Elena interprets this as, *You were right, but you know how Mona is. I think I've calmed her down.*

The patriarch of the family, Alan, is picking at Elena in an attempt to defuse the tension and return the get-together to lighthearted frivolity. Sam, who was the target of Elena's outburst, is feeling annoyance, frustration, and embarrassment. Calmly but directly, he says, "Elena, I'm not sure if everyone agrees with you about not wanting to come to my house for Christmas, but if you don't want to, then please just say so and we can discuss it as a family. It was just an idea I had. I would have enjoyed hosting you all at my house, but I can understand if that's difficult or not the group's consensus. Why doesn't everyone share their ideal plan for celebrating Christmas this year?"

Family Member	Satir Family Communication Style
Elena	
Diana	
Mona	
Rose	
Alan	
Sam	

1. Imagine if no one in the family used a leveling (assertive) communication style. What are the potential short-term and long-term consequences?

____

____

____

____

____

____

Name ____________________ Date ____________ Class ____________

Lesson 3.3 Activity E

Key Terms Review

Part 1

Answer the following questions to review the lesson's key terms.

1. What are airborne chemical messengers released by the body, such as through sweat, that cause reactions from other members of the same species?

2. What is a deep emotional bond between two people characterized by an enduring attraction to each other?

3. What is the ease with which two people can be together?

4. What is the part of your brain where you store all the relevant information about your partner's life?

5. What describes when partners completely withdraw from interacting with each other?

6. What is the perception of closeness to another person that allows for sharing of personal feelings, understanding, affirmation, and demonstration of caring?

7. What is the tendency for one person's negative behavior to instigate another's negative behavior?

Part 2

Review the Five Love Languages in Figure 3.16 and answer the following questions.

1. Which love language do you like to receive the most and why?

2. Which love language do you like to give the most and why?

3. If you send someone a card of encouragement, to which love language does that act relate?

4. Which love language avoids being distracted or unfocused when together?

5. Which love language communicates through nonverbal messages of caring and love?

Name ______________________ Date ____________ Class ____________

Lesson 3.3 Activity F

Setting Boundaries

Review the nine examples from the text of behaviors a partner can practice to build emotional intimacy. Identify which behavior is being highlighted in each example.

1. Juan shares his insecurity about his haircut with his partner.

   ____

2. Sienna giggles when her boyfriend tells a funny story.

   ____

3. Ellie shares that she is upset when her partner does not empty the dishwasher.

   ____

4. Carol thanks her husband for always making her coffee in the morning.

   ____

5. Campbell is telling his girlfriend Suri a story about work. Suri nods her head as she listens and asks questions as he is sharing.

   ____

6. Randel is cheering on his wife as she runs a marathon.

   ____

7. Janelle lets her partner know that she likes the new haircut.

   ____

8. Louis spends quality time with his girlfriend because that is her love language.

   ____

9. Moira discusses the issue of laundry with her spouse, indicating that the laundry is the issue and not her spouse.

   ____

Name ______________________ Date ____________ Class ____________

Chapter 3 Activity G

Chapter Review

Lesson 3.1 Relationship Theories

Match each description with the appropriate dimension of intimacy in relationships:

1. _____ Whether each person influences the other
2. _____ Range of types of interactions between two people
3. _____ How often two people interact
4. _____ Amount of time that two people spend together
5. _____ Significance of the influence between two people

A. frequency of contact
B. duration of contact
C. diversity of different interactions
D. direction of influence
E. strength of influence

Considering the dimensions of intimacy, rank the typical relationships between a young child and the person indicated. 1 = most intimate and 5 = least intimate.

6. _____ Parent/caregiver
7. _____ Teacher
8. _____ Best friend
9. _____ Classmate
10. _____ Sibling

For each statement below, indicate True or False. If False, indicate how the sentence would need to be changed to be considered True.

11. Human beings experience the pain of social rejection in the same ways as they experience physical pain.

____

12. Human beings are not impacted by isolation from others.

____

13. Avoidant attachment styles are prone to fighting, being overly needy, and experiencing hyperarousal and hypervigilance.

____

Lesson 3.2 Family Relationships

For each family, indicate "Yes" if the family is most likely dysfunctional or "No" if the family is not dysfunctional.

1. _____ Jacob feels his family wouldn't notice if he disappeared.
2. _____ The Smiths experience occasional conflict in their family unit.
3. _____ Sara works hard and succeeds at school and in sports because she needs to make the family look good.
4. _____ Trina holds her son close when he comes home from school upset.
5. _____ The Belor parents argue about parenting decisions and authority around their children.

Answer the following questions.

6. _____ Which accurately describes a way in which families function as a system?
   A. Two lowly differentiated people will try to use a third person or thing to disperse the tension.
   B. A child's position among siblings does not impact behavior patterns.
   C. Family members who cut themselves off from the family unit are more differentiated.
   D. Low differentiation is contained within the generation and resets with each future generation.

(Continued)

7. _____ Which family communication style is motivated by finding fault and a fear of alienation and loneliness?
A. Blaming B. Computing C. Distracting D. Placating

8. _____ Which family communication style is motivated by the perception of others and a fear of conflict?
A. Blaming B. Computing C. Leveling D. Placating

9. _____ Which family communication style is *not* motivated by fear?
A. Blaming B. Distracting C. Leveling D. Placating

Lesson 3.3 Romantic Relationships

For each statement, indicate "Yes" or "No" for whether or not it accurately describes love.

1. _____ Love is possessive and controlling.
2. _____ Love is an intimate and deep emotional connection.
3. _____ Love is codependency.
4. _____ Love is the loss of self.
5. _____ Love is maintained through work, care, and attention.

Answer the following questions.

6. _____ The relationship cycle starts with _____.
A. attraction B. commitment C. compatibility D. intimacy

7. _____ As reflected in the walls of the sound relationship house model, a sound relationship is supported by trust and _____.
A. commitment B. love C. communication

8. _____ When frustration, tension, or conflict arises in a relationship, the couple wants to resolve it and return to a place of _____.
A. negativity B. indifference C. positivity

9. _____ When tension presents itself in a sound relationship, the couple turns _____.
A. away from each other B. within themselves C. toward each other

10. _____ Learning about their partner's history, relationships, goals, beliefs, values, and strengths is part of creating a _____.
A. love map B. shared meaning C. self-soothing practice

11. _____ The _____ warning sign of a failing relationship is demonstrated when partners attack each other's character, personality, and identity.
A. criticism B. defensiveness C. contempt

12. _____ Even if they do not agree with their partner's behavior, thoughts, or feelings, _____ couples value empathy and compassion.
A. volatile B. validating C. conflict-avoiding

Name ______________________ Date ______________ Class ______________

CHAPTER 4 Mental Health Throughout the Life Span

Lesson 4.1 Activity A

Key Terms Review

Fill in the blanks in the following statements to review the lesson's key terms.

1. The theory of ______ suggested that learning was an unconscious process in which a conditioned response is achieved through associations between an unconditioned stimulus and neutral stimulus.

   ____

2. ______ is a theory that describes development as the acquisition of learned responses to stimuli.

   ____

3. A person who is unable to imagine situations from someone else's point of view is ______.

   ____

4. The ______ is a law which states that if an association is followed by satisfaction, it will be strengthened, and if it is followed by annoyance, it will be weakened.

   ____

5. A theory that focuses on a person learning behavior by observing people, interactions, and responses in their environment is called ______.

   ____

6. ______ is the process of encouraging a response to a stimulus.

   ____

7. ______ describes engaging in behaviors that promote the well-being of future generations.

   ____

8. Edward Thorndike introduced the theory of ______, or the idea that a person's response could be voluntary and that reward and punishment served as motivating forces to a person's choice.

   ____

9. ______ is the process of discouraging a response to a stimulus.

   ____

10. The realization that an object exists even though it may no longer be visible is called ______.

    ____

11. ______ intervene in the stimulus-response relationship proposed by behaviorists.

    ____

Name ______________________ Date ______________ Class ____________

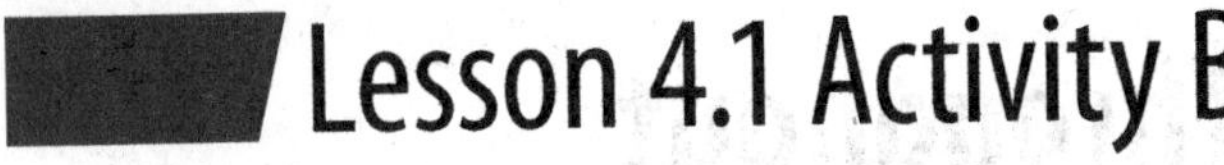

Lesson 4.1 Activity B

Compare Developmental Theories

Complete the table below to develop a graphic organizer that compares developmental theories.

Theory	Behaviorist	Cognitive	Social Learning	Psychosocial
Premise/Short Definition				
Founder(s)				
Principles/ Stages				
Your Personal Thoughts, Criticism, and Questions				

Name ______________________ Date ______________ Class ______________

Lesson 4.2 Activity C

Key Terms Review

Review the lesson's key terms by matching the term with the example.

1. _____ The failure to provide for the basic needs of a person in one's care
2. _____ An educational approach that prioritizes the full scope of a child's developmental needs
3. _____ Internal or external factors that are associated with an increased possibility that a disorder or situation will subsequently develop
4. _____ Interactions in which one person behaves in a cruel, violent, demeaning, or invasive manner toward another person or an animal
5. _____ People who have regular contact with vulnerable people and are legally required to ensure a report is made when abuse is observed or suspected
6. _____ Actions completed in an effort to benefit other individuals or society as a whole
7. _____ A healthy layer of fatty tissue that protects the brain cells and speeds up messages
8. _____ Potentially traumatic events that occur in childhood and adolescence
9. _____ Internal or external factors that decrease the likelihood that a particular disorder or situation will develop
10. _____ Attempts to deal with depression, pain, or intense emotions by using drugs, alcohol, or other substances without the guidance of a doctor
11. _____ Activities that increase insight, empathy, and brain integration
12. _____ The mental picture someone forms of their body as a whole, including its physical characteristics and their attitudes toward these characteristics

A. abuse
B. adverse childhood experiences (ACEs)
C. body image
D. mandated reporters
E. mindsight exercises
F. myelin
G. neglect
H. prosocial behavior
I. protective factors
J. risk factors
K. self-medicating
L. whole child approach

Name ______________________ Date ______________ Class __________

Lesson 4.2 Activity D

Protective Factors versus Risk Factors for ACEs

Part 1

Review the factors described below. Answer with a "P" if it is a Protective Factor and answer with an "R" if it is a Risk Factor.

1. _____ A family member (who was abused) providing care for a child
2. _____ High rate of gun violence in the neighborhood
3. _____ A family that enjoys family outings
4. _____ A strong community center that provides services and resources
5. _____ Low family income
6. _____ Positive group of friends
7. _____ A family that likes to golf together
8. _____ Chronic illness in the family
9. _____ Lack of access to food
10. _____ A focus on school and the importance of school

Part 2

Read the risk factor and suggest a protective factor that would help alleviate the risk.

1. Lack of food in a household

   ____

2. Fear of walking home alone at night

   ____

3. Lack of access to food in the neighborhood

   ____

4. Lack of connection with a caregiver

   ____

5. High conflict in the home

   ____

Name ______________________ Date ____________ Class ____________

Lesson 4.2 Activity E

Reading Charts – Mental Health Treatment for Children

Analyze the table below, then respond to the following questions.

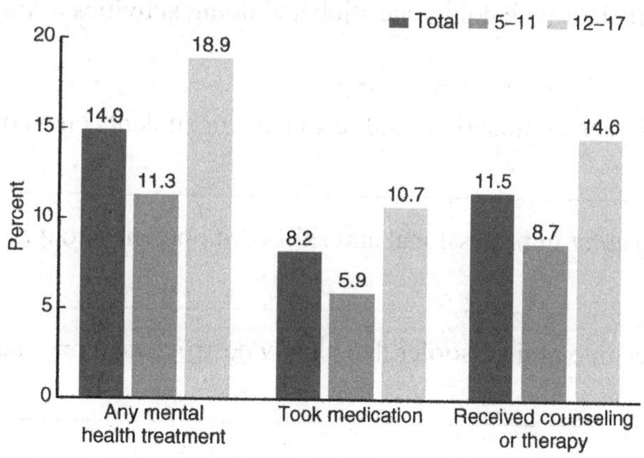

Figure 1. Percentage of children aged 5-17 years who had received any mental health treatment, taken medication for their mental health, or received counseling or therapy from a mental health professional in the past 12 months, by age group. Note that children were considered to have received any mental health treatment if they were reported to have taken medication for their mental health, received counseling or therapy from a mental health professional, or both. Estimates are based on household interviews of a sample of the US civilian noninstitutionalized population in 2021.

1. _____ _____ percent of children aged 5-17 receive some form of mental health treatment.
   A. 8.2 B. 11.5 C. 14.9 D. 18.9
2. _____ Which is an accurate interpretation of the data in the table?
   A. Children aged 12-17 have higher rates of mental illness than 5–11-year-olds.
   B. Children aged 12-17 have lower rates of mental illness than 5–11-year-olds.
   C. Children aged 12-17 receive mental health treatment at higher rates than 5–11-year-olds.
   D. Children aged 12-17 receive mental health treatment at lower rates than 5–11-year-olds.
3. _____ Children aged 5-17 are _____ to receive counseling or therapy treatment than medication treatment for mental health.
   A. more likely B. less likely C. equally likely
4. Describe your reactions to the data. This may include things you found interesting or surprising, questions or wonderings you have about the data, and/or beliefs you may have had that the data confirms.

____

____

____

5. Data is only useful when it helps to share a story. What is the story that this chart is telling?

____

____

____

____

Name ______________________ Date ______________ Class ____________

Lesson 4.3 Activity F

Key Terms Review

Answer the following questions to review the lesson's key terms.

1. What describes spending sufficient time doing one's job and doing activities of one's personal life?

   ____

2. What is a center that provides accommodations and resources for students on a college campus?

   ____

3. What describes a person engaging in professional and skill development throughout their life?

   ____

4. What is a progressive, irreversible brain disorder that slowly destroys memory and thinking skills?

   ____

5. What describes a significant decrease or ending of contact with individuals with whom one formerly had close relationships?

   ____

6. What model describes the essential life skills people learn in parenthood?

   ____

7. What medical condition involves the deterioration of memory, cognitive function, and executive function?

   ____

8. What describes the employment that occurs after leaving a long-term career?

   ____

9. What involves leaving an older adult who needs help alone without planning for their care?

   ____

10. What are activities performed each day, including bathing, medication support, meal preparation, and dressing?

    ____

11. What involves money or belongings being stolen from an older adult?

    ____

Name ______________________________ Date ______________ Class ______________

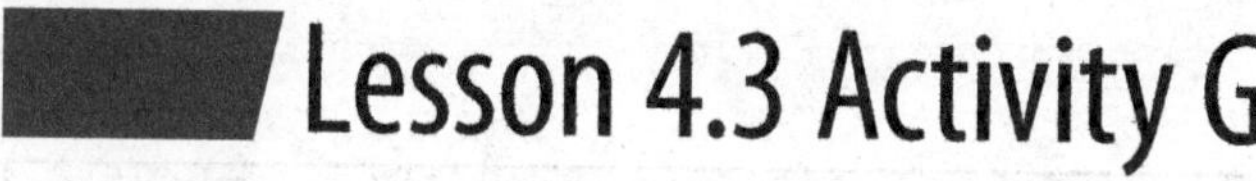

Lesson 4.3 Activity G

Mental Health in Older Adulthood

Select one of the mental health topics for older adults and conduct research on the topic. Record your notes in the space provided below. Then, produce a public service announcement (PSA) video to increase awareness and understanding of the topic. Consider concluding your PSA with a "call to action."

Potential Topics

- Finding meaning in life
- Alzheimer's disease
- Making peace/overcoming resentment
- Elder abuse
- Depression in older adulthood
- Elder financial abuse
- Dementia in older adulthood
- Elder neglect

Research Notes

Notes	Source(s)

(Continued)

PSA Plan

Audio (what viewer will hear)	Visual (what viewer will see)

Name ________________ Date ________ Class ________

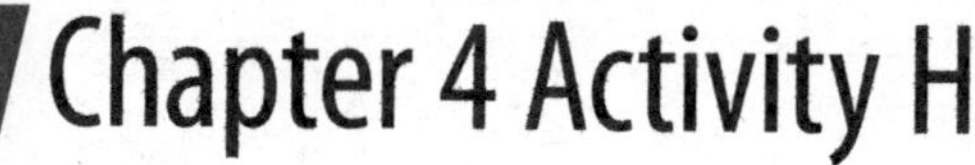

Chapter 4 Activity H

Chapter Review

Lesson 4.1 Theories in Developmental Psychology

Indicate whether each statement is associated with behaviorist (B), cognitive (C), social learning (S), or psychosocial (P) development theories.

1. _____ Scientists should ignore emotions and thoughts and focus on what could be clearly observed.
2. _____ Children go through a stage where they are said to be egocentric, unable to take the perspective of others.
3. _____ Learning is an unconscious process of conditioning responses to a stimulus.
4. _____ Representational play occurs when a child sees a toy as a symbol for a real-life object.
5. _____ There are developmental stages throughout the entire life span.
6. _____ Reproduction addresses the physical ability to reproduce observed behaviors.
7. _____ Observational learning is a foundational principle of this theory.
8. _____ Generativity involves engaging in behaviors that benefit future generations.

Lesson 4.2 Mental Health Issues in Childhood and Adolescence

1. Identify and explain three practices that promote child development.

____

____

____

2. Identify and explain three things that hinder child development.

____

____

____

3. _____ Adolescent brain development is characterized by _____.
   A. the final stage of brain development
   B. an increasingly less integrated brain
   C. a process of generalization
   D. a process of specialization

4. _____ Mindsight exercises increase insight, empathy, and brain _____.
   A. development
   B. disintegration
   C. integration
   D. formation

5. _____ All of the following are mindsight exercises, *except* _____.
   A. positively changing and reframing past memories
   B. practicing independence and testing boundaries
   C. honoring the various parts of your identity
   D. mindfulness, awareness, and breathing

6. _____ What is the relationship between career decision-making and identity?
   A. A person's career contributes to their identity.
   B. A person's career is informed by their identity.
   C. A person's career should be kept separate from their identity.
   D. A person's career contributes to their identity and is informed by their identity.

(Continued)

7. _____ Body acceptance involves reinforcing the belief that _____.
A. all bodies are worthy of love and respect
B. some bodies are good and others are bad
C. dieting and calorie restriction are important skills
D. societal messages about beauty, body size, and worthiness are true

Lesson 4.3 Mental Health Issues in Adulthood

1. Which mental health issues may present themselves to young adults in college?

____

____

____

2. How can college students respond to the mental health issues of college life?

____

____

____

3. _____ In which stage of parenting do parents develop an attachment relationship with the child and adapt to the new baby?
A. Departure B. Interpretive C. Image-making D. Nurturing

4. _____ In which stage of parenting do parents consider what it means to be a parent and plan for changes to accommodate a child?
A. Authority B. Departure C. Image-making D. Interdependent

5. _____ Which response to the question "Where is your child right now?" *best* reflects an authoritarian parenting style?
A. "I don't know. Haven't seen them in a couple days."
B. "They wanted to go to the movies, so that's where they are."
C. "We decided they could go to a friend's house after they finished their chores."
D. "They are at home and will be in their bedroom with the lights out in 20 minutes."

6. _____ Which response to the question "Where is your child right now?" *best* reflects a neglectful parenting style?
A. "I don't know. Haven't seen them in a couple days."
B. "They wanted to go to the movies, so that's where they are."
C. "We decided they could go to a friend's house after they finished their chores."
D. "They are at home and will be in their bedroom with the lights out in 20 minutes."

7. How can adults manage the stress of caregiving for their children and parents while also still working?

____

____

____

8. Identify five risk factors for developing a depressive disorder in older adulthood.

____

____

____

9. What is required for a clinician to diagnose someone with dementia?

____

____

____

Name ______________________ Date ____________ Class ____________

CHAPTER 5 Communities and Mental Health

Lesson 5.1 Activity A

Cultural Conversations

Part 1

For each round in Part 1, discuss the question with your partner and record notes from your partner's response. Follow your teacher's directions for identifying a new partner for each round.

Discussion Questions	Notes of Partner's Responses
Round #1 What was your favorite childhood food? Or a family speciality?	
Round #2 Where did you grow up? How do you think that shaped who you are?	
Round #3 Share a challenging situation or conflict that you later realized may have resulted from a cultural difference (or because of differences in communication styles or word usage).	
Round #4 What is something you realized your family does differently from how others do it?	

(Continued)

Part 2

On your own, reflect on the responses you received and respond to the following debrief questions.

1. What cultural norms emerged in your interview? These may be cultural norms that you recognize about your own cultural identity or those that you may have identified from your partner's responses.

2. What did you find surprising, interesting, or difficult during this activity?

3. Openness, curiosity, and acceptance are important skills for professional helpers. How did you practice these skills during your interviews? How could you improve these skills?

4. Consider culture as a source of strength and resources. In what ways does culture support a person's mental health and well-being?

Name ______________________ Date ____________ Class ____________

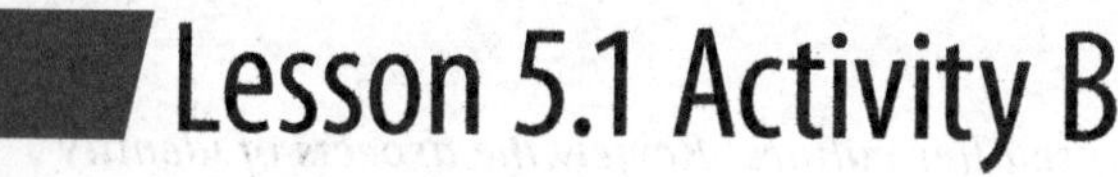

Lesson 5.1 Activity B

Key Terms Review

Part 1

Fill in the blanks in the following statements to review the lesson's key terms.

1. _____ is the ability to influence others even when they try to resist that influence.

 ____

2. _____ are rules, values, or standards of what is considered acceptable and appropriate behavior within a culture.

 ____

3. An enduring social group living in a particular place whose members are mutually interdependent and share political and other institutions, laws, and a common culture is called a(n) _____.

 ____

4. _____ are behaviors that are prohibited or strongly disapproved of within a culture.

 ____

5. Organizations with the belief that all people are equal and deserve equal rights and opportunities are called _____.

 ____

6. _____ is the distinctive customs, values, beliefs, knowledge, art, and language that serve as the basis for everyday behaviors and practices of a society or community.

 ____

7. The hierarchy that encompasses the most powerful people within an organization, society, community, or family is called a(n) _____.

 ____

8. _____ form within the broad, societal culture and around certain aspects of identity, providing a community within which members find connection, support, expression, and purpose.

 ____

9. The process in which a minority group or person begins to resemble or adopt a society's dominant culture is known as _____.

 ____

(Continued)

Part 2

Each of the following contains an example of people within a smaller culture. Review the aspects of identity supported by smaller cultures in Figure 5.5. Identify the aspect of identity in each example of a smaller culture.

1. LeeAnn and Miguel are chapter members of FCCLA.

 ____

2. Eloise and Grace meet at their weekly senior citizens meeting.

 ____

3. Students from the Midwest meet at an annual conference.

 ____

4. Brielle meets with her synagogue's youth group on Wednesday nights.

 ____

5. Edwin and Louise are part of a group advocating for improved accessibility for those with disabilities.

 ____

6. Morah meets her friends at the Latino Community Center.

 ____

Name ______________________ Date ____________ Class ____________

Lesson 5.2 Activity C

Key Terms Review

Review the lesson's key terms by matching the term with the example.

1. _____ The delegation of increased decision-making powers to individuals or groups in a community
2. _____ The extent to which a community believes it has the ability to create change and promote positive behaviors of its members
3. _____ Engages people with one or more common characteristics in working together
4. _____ The strength of relationships and the sense of solidarity among members of a community
5. _____ The extent to which those who are diverse actually feel or are welcomed to participate in the community
6. _____ The fair and equitable division of resources, opportunities, and privileges in society
7. _____ Recognizes that the relationships among people within a community enable it to function effectively
8. _____ The presence of differences among people
9. _____ The promotion of justice, impartiality, and fairness within the procedures, processes, and distribution of resources by communities

A. collective efficacy
B. community
C. diversity
D. empowerment
E. equity
F. inclusion
G. social capital
H. social cohesion
I. social justice

Name ______________________ Date ______________ Class ____________

Lesson 5.2 Activity D

Community Resource Mapping

Professional helpers help clients access and use resources in their community. Some helpers even help build and strengthen communities. Resource mapping is an activity that helpers use to support their work.

Part 1

Working in small groups, brainstorm the resources that you have in your local community. Resources can be very wide-ranging. Consider cultural resources, support services resources, faith-based resources, government resources, education and information resources, environmental and recreational resources, and more.

HINT: When you think you may be finished, try to list 10 more. Repeat this until you can no longer come up with 10 more resources for your list.

Part 2

Within your small group, discuss how each resource supports individuals and families and their mental health. Remember mental health includes cognitive, social, and emotional health. Then discuss the following small group debrief questions. Use the space provided to take your own notes on the discussion.

Question	Discussion Notes
What community strengths emerged as you mapped your community resources?	
If you could implement new resources in your community, what would they be?	

Name ______________________ Date ____________ Class ____________

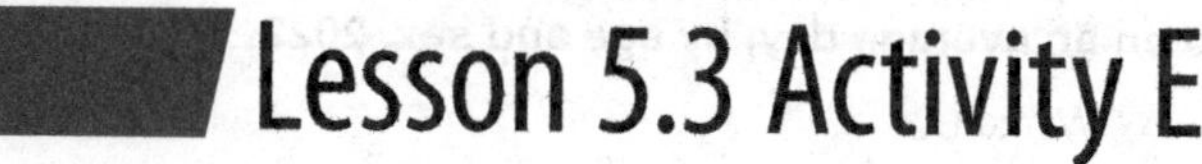

Lesson 5.3 Activity E

Volunteerism Statistics

Review the data on volunteerism and answer the following questions.

Number of Persons and Average Hours Per Day for Participants in Volunteer Activities in 2022		
Activity	**Number of persons on an average day**	**Average hours**
Administrative and support activities	4,712,000	1.56
Social service and care activities	3,187,000	2.23
Attending meetings, conferences, and training	2,038,000	2.15
Participating in performance and cultural activities	721,000	2.40
Indoor and outdoor maintenance, building, and cleanup activities	470,000	2.07

US Bureau of Labor Statistics, 2024

1. Combining the number of people completing an activity and the average hours spent, which activity had the most total volunteer hours on an average day?

____

2. The average value of volunteering is $33.49 per hour. Rounded to the nearest dollar, what is the economic impact of one day of volunteering in the following activities?

   A. Administrative and support activities

   ____

   B. Social service and care activities

   ____

   C. Indoor and outdoor maintenance, building, and cleanup activities

   ____

3. In which category did volunteers spend the most hours on average?

____

____

____

(Continued)

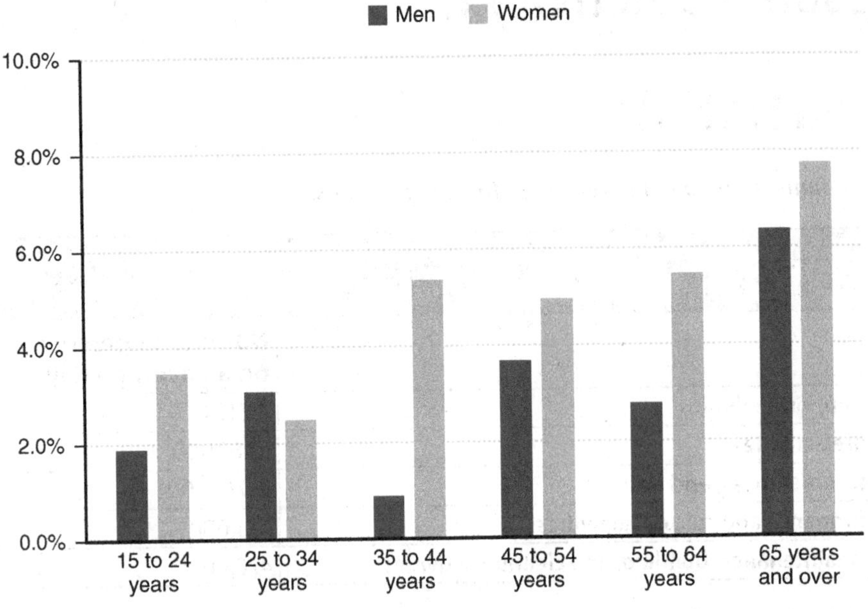

US Bureau of Labor Statistics, 2024

4. Utilizing the chart above, which age group has the largest number of volunteers? What reasons might contribute to higher participation in this age group?

____

____

____

5. What specific groups would benefit from a campaign about the value of volunteering? Include age group and gender. How did you arrive at your answer?

____

____

____

Name ______________________________ Date ______________ Class ______________

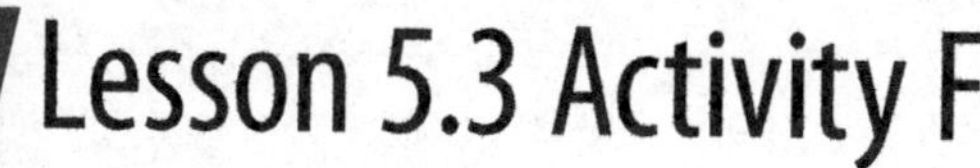

Lesson 5.3 Activity F

Key Terms Review

Part 1

Answer the following questions to review the lesson's key terms.

1. What the government chooses to do, or not do, about a particular issue or problem is called what?

____

2. What is a philosophy that thinks and reflects on moral decisions, especially in difficult situations?

____

3. What includes individual and collective actions that are designed to identify and address issues of public concern?

____

4. What is an activity by an individual or group with the intent to influence decisions within political, economic, and social institutions?

____

5. What occurs when people seek out opportunities to help others in need by making a significant and ongoing commitment to them?

____

6. What are the qualities and behaviors deemed by society to be morally good?

____

7. What is the concept of what is right and wrong, or good and bad, human behavior?

____

8. What is the action of engaging in robust campaigning to affect political or social change?

____

Part 2

Answer the following questions with complete sentences.

1. Describe one instance where you volunteered or would like to volunteer.

____

____

____

2. Review Figure 5.13. What do you see as your personal benefits to volunteering?

____

____

____

Name ____________________ Date ____________ Class ____________

Lesson 5.3 Activity G

Moral Development

For each scenario below, indicate the level of moral development that the individual most likely represents, according to Kohlberg and Gilligan's theories.

1. Trevor does not stay out past his curfew because if he does, his guardians will take away his cell phone for a week.

   ____

2. Sarah focuses all of her time, energy, and attention on meeting the needs of her children.

   ____

3. Martin makes sure he is respectful of teachers and turns in his assignments on time, and he enjoys when his football coach pulls him aside to praise his schoolwork.

   ____

4. Lisa notices that she will get in trouble at her grandmother's house for being loud and rambunctious, but she will not get in trouble with that at her own house.

   ____

5. Javier is arrested for nonviolent civil disobedience, protesting a new law that he believes violates human rights.

   ____

6. Bethany makes time in her busy schedule and sets aside money in her budget to see a mental health therapist to make sure that she is meeting her own needs.

   ____

7. Timmothy is ambitious and wants to do well in school so he can get into his top choice for college, but he gets frustrated when his peers misbehave. He wishes they would see the importance of obeying rules to ensure that students like himself can learn.

   ____

8. Jasmine is a teacher. After class, she asks one of her students why she did not turn in her assignment. Jasmine discovers that the student's father was arrested yesterday, and her mother had to work an evening shift, so the student had to make dinner and take care of her younger siblings. Jasmine told the student she would accept the assignment on Monday without deducting late points.

   ____

9. Mohammad's father says that it is inappropriate to stare at people who may have a disability because it can make them feel uncomfortable.

   ____

10. Eliza takes care at work to follow the rules so she can keep her job and one day get promoted from shift supervisor to manager.

    ____

Name ______________________ Date __________ Class __________

Chapter 5 Activity H

Chapter Review

Lesson 5.1 Society and Culture

For each example, indicate the source of power it demonstrates.

1. "Oh, you can't say those types of things around the coach! That's disrespectful!"

____

2. "If you don't do this for me, then I'm going to tell everyone about that thing you did last summer."

____

3. "No, I didn't ask any questions. My doctor said I needed this operation, so I'm getting it."

____

4. "If I want to get a bonus this year, then I need to impress management with my sales figures."

____

5. "The Chief Finance Officer (CFO) denied my request because they said it was not an allowable expense."

____

6. "The only staff who have access to confidential client records are their current counselor and counseling supervisors."

____

For each statement below, indicate if it is True or False. If False, indicate how the statement should be corrected to make it True.

7. Culture influences people's perspectives of the world and influences human behavior.

____

8. While languages vary among cultures, they have little impact on a person's lived experience.

____

9. Cultural norms are universal and do not vary from one culture to the next.

____

10. Smaller cultures can exist within and among the dominant culture.

____

11. People in cultures that are loose are more likely to focus on avoiding mistakes and monitoring other people's behavior to catch them when they do not conform.

____

(Continued)

Lesson 5.2 Communities

1. _____ Which *best* exemplifies what it means to be a community?
   A. A local tennis store offers fundamentals classes to beginners.
   B. An online science-fiction fan club allows people to post reviews of new books.
   C. Colleagues at work meet weekly to update each other on their individual projects.
   D. A neighborhood works together to support a family whose house was destroyed in a fire.

2. _____ Which community *least likely* exemplifies a healthy community?
   A. Community A offers a high level of social services that focus on ensuring the basic needs of its members are met.
   B. Community B has no worker protections, allowing businesses to exploit community members to increase sales and profit.
   C. Community C prioritizes building and maintaining public schools in their budget.
   D. Community D works to recruit a variety of types of employers, including new and emerging industries.

3. _____ A city requires new housing developments to build a mix of housing options, like large single-family homes, small one-story cottages, duplexes, townhouses, and condos. Plans must also include open spaces for parks and social activities. This promotes which healthy community indicator?
   A. An optimal level of appropriate public health
   B. Access to quality education and job skills training
   C. High-quality environment, including adequate housing
   D. Participation by members in the decisions that affect them personally

4. _____ A town is looking to build a new park. They host in-person and virtual meetings, presenting the design and asking for feedback. This promotes which healthy community indicator?
   A. Transparency and opportunities for interactions among community members and leaders
   B. An optimal level of appropriate public health and equitable access to healthcare services
   C. Access to quality education, job skills training, and employment opportunities
   D. A diverse, vibrant, and innovative economy

5. _____ A community's leaders feel that nothing is changing or improving. What should they do next?
   A. Schedule more meetings.
   B. Limit meetings to a core group.
   C. Invite new members to the conversation.
   D. Bring in an outside group to advise them.

6. _____ A community's leaders are developing a five-year strategic plan. How should they approach this?
   A. Brush failures under the rug.
   B. Focus on what is working and what is possible.
   C. Use an outside firm to conduct a study and develop strategies.
   D. Limit excessive conversation by deciding on the strategies among themselves.

7. _____ A community's leaders invest in social and recreational activities to facilitate connection. Which healthy community principle for leaders does this exemplify?
   A. Humans can handle anything as long as we are together.
   B. Expect leaders to come from anywhere.
   C. Everything is a failure in the middle.
   D. The wisdom resides within us.

(Continued)

Name ______________________________

Match each community building principle to the appropriate example.

8. _____ A community provides free weekly transportation to mental health appointments for members without transportation.

9. _____ After recognizing that nearly all elected officials in the county came from the same racial and ethnic background, despite the population being much more diverse, a county developed a program to recruit members from underrepresented racial and ethnic groups to run for local offices.

10. _____ A community celebrates the various backgrounds of its members through an annual multicultural fair.

11. _____ Upon becoming aware that many of their older adults feel isolated and lonely, the community knows they can fix this and forms a task force to solve this problem.

12. _____ Recognizing that natural disasters are on the rise and that they are increasingly susceptible to property damage, a community works to increase their preparation and resilience. Part of this includes encouraging relationships among its members to make it a more close-knit community that can support one another if disaster strikes.

13. _____ In an effort to bring in new voices and fresh ideas to the conversation and support the civic engagement of young people, a community creates a youth budget council that controls a portion of the community's budget and provides feedback on other budgetary decisions.

A. collective efficacy
B. diversity
C. equity
D. empowerment
E. inclusion
F. social cohesion and capital

Lesson 5.3 Civic Engagement and Moral Development

1. _____ Which is *not* an example of civic engagement?
   A. Researching and learning about current events and issues
   B. Volunteering to clean up a park or green space
   C. Voting in local, state, and national elections
   D. Going to work and keeping a job

2. _____ Since his mother passed away from breast cancer, Jason has started volunteering at fundraising events for breast cancer research. This exemplifies which mental health benefit of volunteering?
   A. Cognitive exercise
   B. Improves confidence
   C. Processing grief
   D. Stress reduction

3. _____ Since volunteering for Habitat for Humanity, Tre has learned a whole new set of construction skills and abilities. This exemplifies which mental health benefit of volunteering?
   A. Cognitive exercise
   B. Improves confidence
   C. Meaning-making
   D. Prevents feeling isolated

4. _____ Since volunteering with a community service group, Jasmine has noticed that her overall mood has become more hopeful, positive, and calm. This exemplifies which mental health benefit of volunteering?
   A. Cognitive exercise
   B. Discover and explore passions
   C. Process grief
   D. Promote joy

(Continued)

For each statement below, indicate if it is True or False. If False, indicate how the statement can be adjusted to make it True.

5. Public policy is the result of decisions made by legislators alone.

____

6. Professional helpers rarely engage in advocacy work to bring about improvements in the systems within which people live, work, and seek treatment.

____

7. To ensure their activism is effective, social movements can focus on creating a friendly, inviting, and passionate environment; mobilizing or coordinating frequent events or campaigns to keep attention on their issue; and choosing nonviolent tactics.

____

8. The qualities or behaviors deemed by society to be morally good are called virtues.

____

9. Gilligan modified Kohlberg's theory of moral development to reflect a lower valuation of personal relationships.

____

10. Understanding that universal ethical principles are more important than law or social order is characteristic of conventional morality.

____

11. According to Gilligan, women's postconventional morality is characterized by the virtue of nonviolence.

____

12. Some psychologists argue that Gilligan's theory elevates the role of caregiver above other roles women can assume.

____

Name ______________________ Date ____________ Class ____________

CHAPTER 6

The Biology of Psychology

Lesson 6.1 Activity A

Key Terms Review

Fill in the blanks in the following statements to review the lesson's key terms.

1. The fundamental cells of the nervous system are called _____.

 ____

2. _____ branch out from the soma and are responsible for receiving signals.

 ____

3. The body system which includes a set of glands that secrete hormones into the bloodstream is the _____.

 ____

4. _____ is the sense of self-movement, force, and body position within a person's environment.

 ____

5. The long fiber that transmits electrical impulses away from the soma to other cells is called _____.

 ____

6. The body system that guides messages to and from the central nervous system is called the _____.

 ____

7. Chemical messengers from one neuron to the next are called _____.

 ____

8. _____ provide support, nutrition, and insulation to neurons and help neurons with signal transmission.

 ____

9. _____ are contact points between neurons, where axons meet dendrites.

 ____

10. _____ is a process where molecules within and surrounding the axon membrane send an electrical impulse down the axon to the axon terminals.

 ____

11. _____ are the physical, mental, and behavioral changes that follow a 24-hour cycle.

 ____

12. _____ is the hormone connected to the feelings of trust and social bonding.

 ____

Name ______________________________ Date ______________ Class __________

Lesson 6.1 Activity B

The Nervous System

Part 1

Match each nervous system component with its description.

1. _____ Consists of the brain and the spinal column
2. _____ Triggers a call to action in response to stimulation
3. _____ Regulates, or calms, the sympathetic nervous system
4. _____ Transmits impulses toward the central nervous system
5. _____ Transmits impulses away from the central nervous system
6. _____ All parts of the nervous system, except the brain and spinal column
7. _____ Made up of nerves that transmit signals to vital organs, mediating unconscious motor output
8. _____ Made up of nerves that transmit signals to the skin and muscles and involves conscious motor output

A. autonomic nervous system
B. central nervous system
C. motor division
D. parasympathetic nervous system
E. peripheral nervous system
F. sensory division
G. somatic nervous system
H. sympathetic nervous system

Part 2

Label the components of the peripheral nervous system organization chart below.

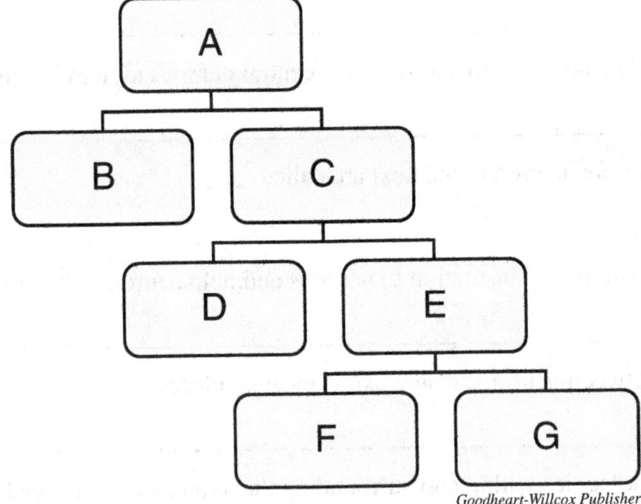

A. ______________________________

B. ______________________________

C. ______________________________

D. ______________________________

E. ______________________________

F. ______________________________

G. ______________________________

Name ______________________ Date ______________ Class ______________

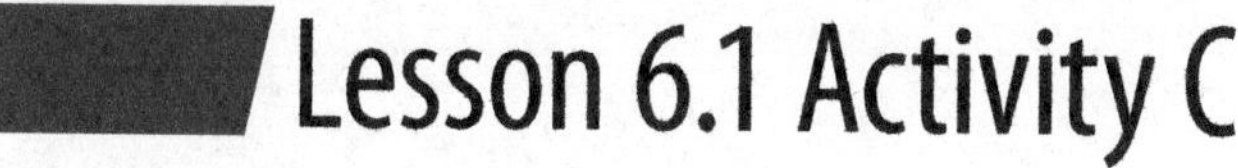

Lesson 6.1 Activity C

Neurotransmitter Research

Record the neurotransmitter you have been assigned below. Then use the graphic organizer to record notes from researching the neurotransmitter. Finally, develop a short presentation using the media or formats allowed by your teacher.

Prompt	Response
Neurotransmitter	
Role(s) and Effect(s)	
Mental/Physical Disorder Associations	
Related Medications	
Other Interesting or Important Facts	

Name ______________________ Date ______________ Class ____________

Lesson 6.2 Activity D

Key Terms Review

Review the lesson's key terms by matching the term with the example.

1. _____ A cluster of several brain structures located between the left and right hemispheres of the outer brain
2. _____ A narrow network of neurons running through the medulla and pons that enables the body to sleep, walk, eat, and feel pain
3. _____ A cluster of nuclei that are responsible for motor function and motor learning, executive functions and behavior, and emotions
4. _____ The process of producing images of the structure or activity of the brain or other parts of the nervous system
5. _____ A layer of 20 billion interconnected neurons that cover the cerebrum
6. _____ A pair of egg-shaped structures that receive sensory information related to seeing, hearing, touching, and tasting
7. _____ A baseball-sized structure of the brain that is responsible for nonverbal learning, memory, regulating emotions, and voluntary movement
8. _____ Two lima-bean-sized clusters of neurons involved in emotions and memory consolidation
9. _____ Areas in the prefrontal cortex that are related to higher-level cognitive functions like remembering, thinking, learning, and speaking
10. _____ A brain structure that regulates body temperature, circadian rhythms, and hunger
11. _____ A brain structure that is central to learning, memory, and spatial memory
12. _____ An arch-shaped structure just below the outer brain that coordinates sensory input with emotions
13. _____ A brain structure located behind the forehead that is responsible for judging processes like decision-making and planning
14. _____ A brain structure divided into two hemispheres, which is responsible for the integration of complex sensory and neural functions
15. _____ A thick bundle of nerves that connects the left and right hemispheres of the cerebrum

A. amygdala
B. association areas
C. basal ganglia
D. cerebral cortex
E. cerebellum
F. cerebrum
G. cingulate cortex
H. corpus callosum
I. hippocampus
J. hypothalamus
K. limbic system
L. neuroimaging
M. prefrontal cortex
N. reticular formation
O. thalamus

Name ______________________ Date ____________ Class ____________

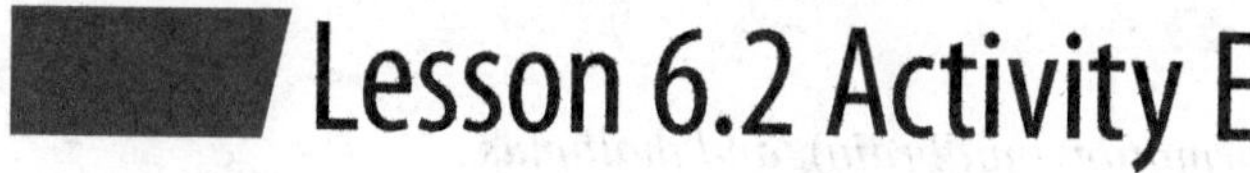

Lesson 6.2 Activity E

Structure and Function

Part 1

In your own words, write a short description of the function of each brain structure.

Brain Structure	Function
Medulla	
Pons	
Reticular Formation	
Thalamus	
Cerebellum	
Amygdala	
Hypothalamus	
Hippocampus	
Basal Ganglia	
Cingulate Cortex	
Cerebrum	
Corpus Callosum	
Cerebral Cortex	
Frontal Lobe	
Parietal Lobe	
Occipital Lobe	
Temporal Lobe	
Prefrontal Cortex	
Association Areas	

(Continued)

Part 2

Label the diagram below with the medulla, pons, reticular formation (midbrain), and thalamus.

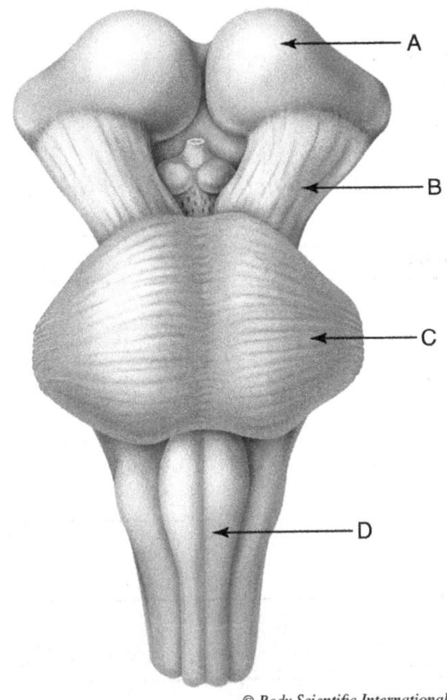

© *Body Scientific International*

A. ______________________________

B. ______________________________

C. ______________________________

D. ______________________________

Part 3

Label the diagram below with the lobes of the cerebral cortex.

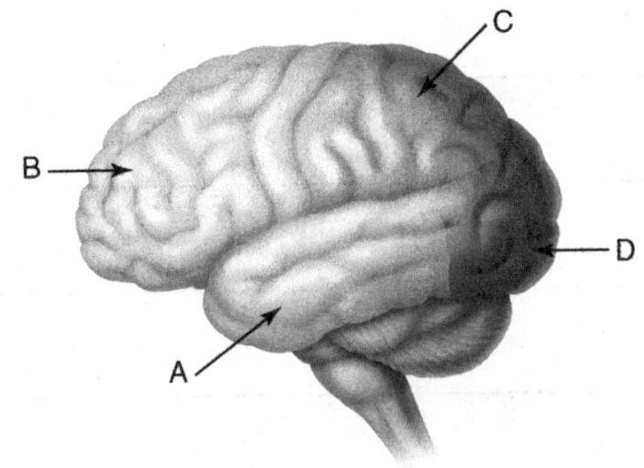

VectorMine/Shutterstock.com

A. ______________________________

B. ______________________________

C. ______________________________

D. ______________________________

Name ______________________ Date ______________ Class ______________

Lesson 6.3 Activity F

Key Terms Review

Answer the following questions to review the lesson's key terms.

1. What is a process where the brain organizes and interprets sensory information and puts it into context?

   ____

2. What describes the process where people become "immune" to a sensation that they have experienced for some time?

   ____

3. What is a process where the senses receive information, relying on outside stimuli?

   ____

4. What is the tendency to see familiar objects as having a standard shape, size, color, or location regardless of changes in the viewing angle, distance, motion, or lighting?

   ____

5. What contains six principles for how the brain speeds up processing all the stimuli it is responsible for integrating?

   ____

6. What describes the influence of a variety of psychological factors on the perception of one's environment?

   ____

7. What is the minimum stimulation needed to register a particular stimulus half of the time?

   ____

8. What describes the eyes relaying a two-dimensional image and the brain taking that data and determining which objects are closer and which are farther away?

   ____

9. What describes how different two stimuli need to be for the brain to recognize them as different 50 percent of the time?

   ____

10. What theory predicts how and when a person will detect weak stimuli?

    ____

11. What is the brain's ability to take a two-dimensional image from the eyes and determine how fast and in which direction elements are moving?

    ____

12. What is the complex task of deciphering shapes and their relationship to one another?

    ____

Name ______________________ Date ______________ Class ____________

Lesson 6.3 Activity G

Sensation and Perception Scenarios

Using the principles of sensation and perception described in Lesson 6.3, explain in psychological terms what is happening in the following scenarios.

1. Javier works in a residential care facility. As he is walking around, he likes to greet residents. He has noticed that with some residents, he needs to speak more loudly for them to notice and hear him. But for other residents, speaking too loudly seems to be distressing. He keeps a mental note of the volume he should use when greeting each resident.

____

____

____

____

____

2. Jasmine has been on so many bad first dates lately. She reluctantly gets ready and orders a ride to go meet her date at The Optimist Coffee Shop at 10:00 a.m. On the way, she thinks, "What's the point?" During the date, Jasmine is bored, and finds her date unattractive and the coffee lackluster.

   Meanwhile, Jessica is newly divorced from an unhappy marriage and has taken some time to go to therapy and process her feelings about the relationship. She is ready to get back out there and start dating. She has her first date at The Optimist Coffee Shop this morning. While getting ready, she is having fun putting on clothes that make her feel good and is excited to meet someone new. During the date, Jessica has a good time, finds her date interesting, and comments on how good the coffee tastes.

____

____

____

____

____

3. A police officer is interviewing two witnesses to a bank robbery. Below are the police officer's notes from their interviews.

Witness A	Witness B
• Robber wore all black (long-sleeve shirt and pants) black shoes, full-coverage hood/mask • Robber was tall, like 6'4" • "Dark skin" (hands); asked about gloves, said that the suspect was not wearing gloves	• Robber had black pants, dark brown sweater, gloves, a full-coverage hood/mask, and gray tennis shoes • Robber was kinda tall like, like 6' • Could not see skin; asked about hands, reiterated the suspect wore gloves

Hint: Consider Gestalt psychology laws.

____

____

____

____

____

Name ________________________ Date ____________ Class ____________

Chapter 6 Activity H

Chapter Review

Lesson 6.1 Chemical Messengers

For each of the statements below indicate if it is True or False. If False, indicate how the statement should be corrected to make it True.

1. The nervous system facilitates a process of sensory input, proprioception, and motor output.

____

2. Integration is the process of interpreting and deciding what to do with that information.

____

3. The motor division transmits impulses toward the central nervous system. The sensory division transmits impulses from the central nervous system to the rest of the body.

____

4. Your heartbeat increasing in response to a perceived threat or cardiovascular exercise is an example of a somatic nervous system response.

____

5. A member of the armed forces in a high stress combat situation uses a breathing technique to calm down. The deep breathing technique engages their parasympathetic system.

____

Use the figure of a neuron below to answer questions 6-9.

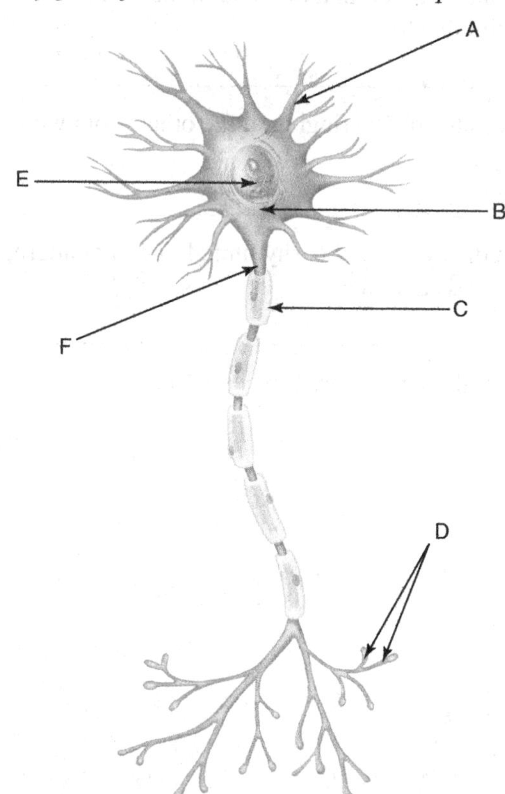

© *Body Scientific International*

6. _____ Which part is responsible for receiving signals?
   A. A
   B. B
   C. E
   D. F

7. _____ Which part is responsible for transmitting electrical impulses away from the soma to other cells?
   A. A
   B. B
   C. E
   D. F

8. _____ At which part are neurotransmitters released?
   A. B
   B. C
   C. D
   D. F

9. _____ Which part accelerates the speed of electrical impulses?
   A. B
   B. C
   C. D
   D. F

(Continued)

Lesson 6.2 The Brain

Indicate if each statement is True or False. If False, describe how the statement could be changed to make it True.

1. For much of human history, the brain was favored as the center of human consciousness.

____

2. People can be either right-brain dominant or left-brain dominant, meaning their brain is predisposed to be more artistic or more mathematical.

____

3. The brain is the organ, while the mind refers to what people experience as a result of what the brain does.

____

For the questions below, select the best answer choice from the options.

4. _____ Which part of the brain is responsible for controlling voluntary movement and is highly susceptible to alcohol?
   A. Amygdala B. Cerebellum C. Corpus callosum D. Medulla

5. _____ What is the name for the outermost layer of the brain, characterized by deep grooves and folds, increasing the surface area to allow for more neurons and glial cells?
   A. Amygdala B. Basal ganglia C. Cerebral cortex D. Hippocampus

6. _____ Which part of the brain continues to develop into a person's 20s and is responsible for executive functioning skills like decision-making and planning?
   A. Cerebral cortex B. Cingulate cortex C. Hypothalamus D. Prefrontal cortex

7. _____ Which lobe of the cerebral cortex is responsible for speaking, abstract thinking, and aspects of one's personality?
   A. Frontal B. Occipital C. Parietal D. Temporal

Lesson 6.3 Sensing and Perceiving

Fill in the blank to answer the following questions.

1. Megan comes over to Trina's house for dinner and points out a musty smell that turns out to be mold behind the wall from a slow water leak. Trina may not have noticed the smell due to _____.

____

2. While waiting for an important call from his doctor, Andy notices his phone ringing in the other room while he's taking a shower. Andy probably noticed the ring due to the _____.

____

3. _____, or engaging both hemispheres of the brain in a visual, auditory, or tactile, rhythmic left-right pattern, can be used to decrease emotional distress and treat post-traumatic stress disorder.

____

4. _____ can be formed where they did not exist before, they can be altered, or they can cease to exist.

____

Label each principle of Gestalt psychology presented below.

Goodheart-Willcox Publisher

Goodheart-Willcox Publisher

Goodheart-Willcox Publisher

Goodheart-Willcox Publisher

5. _______________ 6. _______________ 7. _______________ 8. _______________

Name ______________________ Date ______________ Class ______________

CHAPTER 7 Language and Learning

Lesson 7.1 Activity A

Key Terms Review

Fill in the blanks in the following statements to review the lesson's key terms.

1. _____ is the set of rules and processes that govern sentence structure in a language.

   ____

2. _____ describes a person who can read and write proficiently in two languages.

   ____

3. The region that controls the fine motor functions associated with speech production is called _____.

   ____

4. _____ is a system that combines symbols, sounds, meanings, and rules to allow for communication.

   ____

5. _____ is the study and classification of speech sounds.

   ____

6. _____ describes a person who can speak fluently in more than two languages.

   ____

7. The smallest units of spoken language are called _____.

   ____

8. The words used in phrases and sentences to help a person understand a new word are called _____.

   ____

9. The smallest units of written language are called _____.

   ____

10. _____ describes a person who can speak fluently in two languages.

    ____

11. _____ refers to the application of evidence-based reading instruction practices that promote the development of language, phonological and phonemic awareness, phonics and spelling, fluency, vocabulary, oral language, and comprehension.

    ____

12. _____ is responsible for the understanding of language, by allowing people to process the sounds and symbols that sensory receptors in their eyes and ears relay to the brain.

    ____

Name ______________________ Date ______________ Class ______________

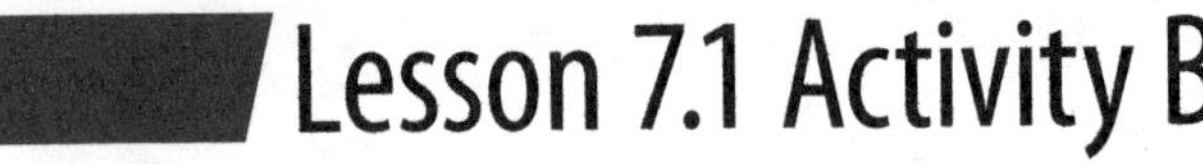

Lesson 7.1 Activity B

Promoting Early Language Learning

Imagine you are an educational psychologist. Use the early language learning principles covered in Lesson 7.1 to develop a training plan for new parents on how to support their child's cognitive development. Create a 45-minute training using the template below.

By the end of the training, what training objectives are you hoping participants will have achieved?

____

____

Training Part	Time	Activity	Resources/Materials
Appetizer: short opener activity that builds interest and activates prior knowledge			
Entrée: lecture-style presentation limited to 10-15 minutes, engaging activity to apply concepts			
Dessert: brief learning check (assessment) and opportunity for reflection			

Name ______________________ Date ______________ Class ______________

Lesson 7.2 Activity C

Key Terms Review

Review the lesson's key terms by matching the term with the example.

1. _____ The type of memory that has immense storage capacity and can be stored indefinitely
2. _____ The retention of information independent of conscious recollection
3. _____ Processing information involuntarily or without conscious intention or control
4. _____ The process of converting sensory input into meaningful information
5. _____ Organizing items into manageable units
6. _____ The short-term storage and manipulation of perceptual and linguistic information
7. _____ The brain's unconscious use of cues to retrieve memory
8. _____ The facts and experiences that one can consciously know and declare
9. _____ Hints and techniques that people use to remember something
10. _____ The gradual fading away of information that has been stored in the brain
11. _____ Memory aids that help with information retention or retrieval
12. _____ Encoding information semantically by giving it meaning and associating it with other information
13. _____ When a person incorporates misleading information into their memory of an event
14. _____ Encoding information on basic auditory or visual levels based on the sound, structure, or appearance of a word

A. automatic processing
B. chunking
C. deep processing
D. explicit memory
E. implicit memory
F. long-term memory
G. misinformation effect
H. mnemonics
I. priming
J. retrieval cues
K. semantic encoding
L. shallow processing
M. storage decay
N. working memory

Name ______________________ Date ____________ Class ________

Lesson 7.2 Activity D

Memory Process Graphic Organizer

Complete the graphic organizer below by summarizing your own explanation of the memory process indicated and then providing your own example of the memory process.

Encoding		
Type	**Explanation**	**Example**
Visual		
Acoustic		
Tactile		
Semantic		

Storage		
Type	**Explanation**	**Example**
Working		
Long-term		
Explicit		
Implicit		

Retrieval		
Type	**Explanation**	**Example**
Recall		
Recognition		
Relearning		

Name ______________________ Date ____________ Class ____________

Lesson 7.3 Activity E

Key Terms Review

Answer the following questions to review the lesson's key terms.

1. What describes the range of things that can be learned with the help of others?

____

2. What describes all forms of knowing and awareness, such as perceiving, conceiving, remembering, reasoning, judging, imagining, and problem-solving?

____

3. What is the branch of psychology that focuses on the measurement of mental attributes, behavior, and performance?

____

4. What involves changing existing concepts and schemas to integrate new information?

____

5. What is a teaching style that supports and facilitates the learner as they learn a new skill or concept, gradually removing those supports as the learner develops mastery?

____

6. What is the awareness of one's own cognitive processes?

____

7. What are collections of basic knowledge about a concept or entity that serve as a guide to perception, interpretation, imagination, or problem-solving?

____

8. What describes the distortion of assessment results, in which a certain group of people were favored to perform well on the assessment?

____

9. What keeps existing concepts and schemas in place while adding new information?

____

10. What refers to the top three processes in the hierarchy of Revised Bloom's Taxonomy?

____

11. What is a general intelligence and broad mental capacity that influences cognitive performance?

____

12. What is the proactive part of motivation that connects knowledge, drive, desire, and instinct?

____

Name ______________________________ Date ______________ Class ____________

Lesson 7.3 Activity F

Divergent Thinking Exercise

Part 1

Using a mental health subject or issue provided by your teacher, take a walk around your home, school, workplace, or surroundings. Take at least five pictures of objects or visual scenes that could be a metaphor for your subject or issue. For each picture, write a description of the metaphor (how the picture relates to or symbolizes the subject or issue).

Picture	Metaphor Description
1	
2	
3	
4	
5	

Part 2

Then, within a small group who has the same topic, create a virtual or physical photo gallery of your pictures and descriptions. Tour the photo gallery and then brainstorm ideas, insights, or solutions from the visual metaphors.

Name _______________ Date _______________ Class _______________

Lesson 7.3 Activity G

Gardner's Theory of Multiple Intelligences

Match the examples with the type of intelligence from Gardner's theory of multiple intelligences involved.

1. _____ Brian determines the structure that will fit into a closet space and builds it to make the best use of space available.
2. _____ Aileen is an avid hiker and knows how to avoid poisonous plants.
3. _____ Sylvia is preparing for a trip to Italy. She is already fluent in English and Spanish and spends a few months prior building her skills in Italian.
4. _____ Marcus has been working really hard on a project. He knows that he can be overstressed and schedules a day off to rest and do something he enjoys.
5. _____ Madison is considering buying a car. There are two cars that are of interest with varying interest rates to purchase. Madison uses her skills to evaluate the costs of the cars by reviewing both the monthly expenses and the overall total cost.
6. _____ Aaron is a consultant working on a long-term project for a tech company. Aaron uses his knowledge of the team members at the tech company to prepare his presentations.
7. _____ Fisher is working on an end-of-year slideshow. The slideshow is very moving and memorable because of the music he uses.
8. _____ Shanice is looking at a career in physical therapy because she enjoys working with people to build strength and heal.

A. Bodily-kinesthetic
B. Interpersonal
C. Verbal-linguistic
D. Logical-mathematical
E. Naturalistic
F. Intrapersonal
G. Visual-spatial
H. Musical

Name ______________________ Date ______________ Class ____________

Chapter 7 Activity H

Chapter Review

Lesson 7.1 Language

For each statement, indicate if it is True or False. If False, indicate how to correct the statement to make it True.

1. Language is essentially a pattern of sounds that brains establish.

____

2. The word "uneventfulness" has three morphemes.

____

3. Clauses consist of a subject (what one is talking about) and a predicate (information about that subject).

____

4. Broca's area allows people to process the sounds and symbols that sensory receptors in their ears and eyes are relaying to the brain into comprehensible morphemes, phrases, and sentences.

____

5. Children can effectively learn language through phones and tablets.

____

6. Language development in the brain peaks from birth to age five.

____

7. Children are learning words even when they cannot say them yet.

____

8. A child who lacks early exposure to language can make up for it eventually.

____

9. Around age five, a new word can be learned by understanding the other words used with it in phrases and sentences.

____

10. Neuroscientific findings suggest that a developed prefrontal cortex is very helpful in language development.

____

11. Being bilingual or multilingual builds the ability to focus, remember, and make decisions.

____

12. Science of Reading is founded on research conducted in the fields of developmental psychology, educational psychology, cognitive science, and cognitive neuroscience.

____

Lesson 7.2 Memory

1. _____ Memory includes all of the following *except* _____.
   A. interpretation of context clues
   B. retention across an interval of time
   C. mental processes of learning or encoding
   D. retrieval or reactivation of the memory

(Continued)

Name ____________________

2. _____ When Robbie notices she is feeling anxious, she closes her eyes and imagines the feeling of warm, wet beach sand between her toes and calms down. Her ability to do this relies on _____.
A. acoustic encoding
B. semantic encoding
C. tactile encoding
D. visual encoding

3. _____ When a sensory memory is encoded with meaning, it is encoded _____.
A. acoustically
B. semantically
C. tactilely
D. visually

4. _____ Which statement *best* characterizes working memory?
A. Working memory retains one to four pieces of information for up to 30 seconds.
B. Working memory retains five to nine pieces of information for up to 30 seconds.
C. Working memory retains ten to fourteen pieces of information for up to 60 seconds.
D. Working memory retains fifteen to nineteen pieces of information for up to 60 seconds.

5. _____ One function of working memory is the central executive, which _____.
A. determines which stimuli are worth your attention
B. temporarily manipulates and stores visual and spatial information
C. temporarily manipulates and stores written and spoken information
D. binds information together about the same event to create a mental representation

6. _____ Knowing how to read is an example of _____ memory.
A. autobiographical
B. episodic
C. semantic
D. procedural

7. _____ Selecting the correct answer choice on a multiple-choice question uses which retrieval process?
A. Recall
B. Recognition
C. Rehearsal
D. Relearning

8. _____ Retracing your steps is an example of _____.
A. mnemonics
B. rehearsal
C. priming
D. storage decay

9. _____ What is one of the most effective methods for retrieving information from long-term memory and involves encoding it semantically?
A. Deep processing
B. Chunking
C. Mnemonics
D. Retrieval cues

10. _____ Researchers have found that about _____ percent of the details in an episodic memory change in a year.
A. 10
B. 25
C. 50
D. 75

11. _____ Which *best* characterizes memory?
A. Memory is an accurate, detailed account of past events.
B. Memory is most similar to information stored in a filing cabinet.
C. Memory is a projection of others' experiences and perspectives.
D. Memory is both a reconstruction and a reproduction of past events.

12. _____ When memory encounters gaps in information, it relies on _____.
A. acronyms
B. chunking
C. patterns
D. shallow processing

13. _____ Memory may serve to support the mind's ability to _____.
A. maintain precise representations of previous events
B. attract romantic partners for the survival of the human species
C. learn and acquire implicit memories that support automatic processing
D. imagine the future, troubleshoot problems, and anticipate what will happen

Lesson 7.3 Cognition and Motivation

1. _____ Cognition describes the parts of the mind that are involved with _____.
A. thinking processes
B. feelings and emotions
C. connection with a higher power
D. maintaining autonomic functions

(Continued)

2. _____ Which characterizes the sociocultural theory of cognitive development?
A. Knowledge is constructed through social interactions.
B. Knowledge is a series of learned responses to stimuli.
C. Language and culture have little influence on learning.
D. Learning depends on strict age-defined developmental stages.

3. _____ A helper is working with a caregiver who gets frustrated with their 16-month-old child for wetting themselves during the day. The helper explains the benefits of making the expectation more realistic and increasing the goal over time between accidents. This *best* exemplifies _____.
A. accommodation
B. assimilation
C. schemas
D. zone of proximal development

4. _____ A helper is working with a client with an eating disorder. When asked what they think of their body, they list all of the things that they do not like. Through therapy, the client comes to recognize the things they like about their body, including how it enables them to do things they enjoy. Which cognitive process *most likely* occurred?
A. The client improved abstraction of their body.
B. The client set boundaries with people who were critical of their body.
C. The client used diet and exercise to achieve an improved body image.
D. The client deprogrammed societal messages around body shape and worthiness.

5. _____ Which cognitive process is considered a higher-order thinking skill?
A. Apply
B. Evaluate
C. Remember
D. Understand

6. _____ Which *best* characterizes conation?
A. One's emotional experience
B. One's assimilation of new schemas
C. One's internal drive to do something
D. One's ability to reason and problem-solve

Answer the following short answer questions.

7. What theory suggests there is a universal skill and knowledge set to which people have varying levels?

_____

8. What view of intelligence encapsulates a person's ability to understand and manage the emotions of themselves and others, relate to others, and use emotions to communicate?

_____

9. What are two criticisms of Gardner's theory of multiple intelligences?

_____

_____

_____

10. What are the three areas of intelligence as suggested by the triarchic theory of intelligence?

_____

11. What five factors contribute to divergent thinking?

_____

_____

12. Explain the difference between reliability and validity in assessment.

_____

_____

_____

13. What term describes the brain's ability to form and reorganize synaptic connections throughout a person's entire life?

_____

Name ______________________ Date ____________ Class ____________

CHAPTER 8 Neurodivergence

Lesson 8.1 Activity A

Special Educator Interview

Working with a partner, interview a special education professional (Part 1). Then, discuss with your partner the responses you received and summarize your findings in an article (Part 2).

Part 1: Special Education Interview

Use the questions below as a starting place, but you may need to ask clarifying questions. Additionally, generate at least 5 additional open-ended questions. Consider questions that will help you understand concepts from the text more deeply.

Prompt	Response
Interviewer(s)	
Interviewee(s)	
Date of Interview	
Start/End Time	
Interview Location	
What is your position or job title?	
Please describe what you do in your role.	
What do you see as the role of special education?	
What challenges do you encounter in your work? What benefits?	
What strengths do you see in your students with disabilities?	
Can you explain the process of creating, updating, and implementing an IEP?	

(Continued)

Open-Ended Question #1:	
Open-Ended Question #2:	
Open-Ended Question #3:	
Open-Ended Question #4:	
Open-Ended Question #5:	

Part 2: Reflection and Summary

Collaborate with your partner to compare notes from the interview and write an article summarizing the interview. Record any additional notes from this collaboration below. Record your article summarizing the interview separately. The article should be between 350 and 500 words.

Name ______________________ Date ____________ Class ____________

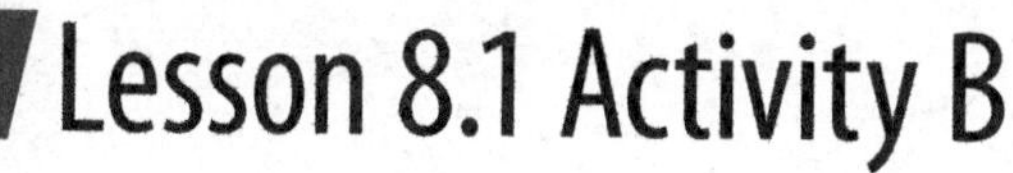

Lesson 8.1 Activity B

Key Terms Review

Fill in the blanks in the following statements to review the lesson's key terms.

1. Displaying atypical neurological patterns of thought or behavior is called _____.

    ____

2. _____ is a specialized area that focuses on providing individualized support and instruction tailored to students with disabilities or exceptionalities.

    ____

3. _____ are changes to the curriculum or instructional resources to meet the needs of students with disabilities.

    ____

4. A(n) _____ is any condition characterized by cognitive and emotional disturbances, abnormal behaviors, impaired functioning, or any combination of these.

    ____

5. _____ is when a person with a disability, as effectively and easily as a person without a disability, can acquire the same information, engage in the same interactions, and enjoy the same services.

    ____

6. _____ is the effort for a child with disabilities, to the greatest extent possible, to be educated alongside children who do not have disabilities.

    ____

7. A(n) _____ is a legally binding document outlining accommodations, modifications, support services, aides progress data, and goals for students with disabilities.

    ____

8. Treating a client, condition, or symptom as psychologically abnormal or unhealthy is called _____.

    ____

9. An approach to improve teaching and learning for all students by setting clear, rigorous goals; anticipating barriers; and proactively designing to minimize those barriers is called _____.

    ____

10. Displaying typical neurological patterns of thought or behavior is called _____.

    ____

11. _____ are changes to the way a student with disabilities is taught or assessed, participates in class, or completes assignments.

    ____

12. _____ is the idea that addressing disadvantages or exclusions for one group of people, like people with disabilities, creates a more effective and accessible environment for everyone.

    ____

13. The _____ is a federal law that guarantees the right to free appropriate education and services to children with disabilities.

    ____

Name ____________________ Date ____________ Class ________

Lesson 8.2 Activity C

Key Terms Review

Review the lesson's key terms by matching the term with the example.

1. _____ Learning disability characterized by language difficulty or delayed language acquisition believed to be association with brain damage or a lag in cerebral maturation
2. _____ The cognitive ability to plan, prioritize, and sustain effort toward a goal, including inhibiting impulse behavior
3. _____ Learning disability that includes cognitive difficulty with mathematics
4. _____ An auditory processing disorder where people have trouble putting meaning to the sound groups that make up words, phrases, and stories
5. _____ A behavioral syndrome characterized by difficulty paying attention, difficulty controlling impulsive behaviors, or being overly active
6. _____ Learning disability characterized by trouble reading, writing, and spelling as a result of cognitive difficulty processing words and letters
7. _____ When a person experiences severe emotional pain because of a failure or feeling rejected
8. _____ Learning disability that includes cognitive difficulty with writing or handwriting, often due to fine motor skill issues
9. _____ When a person has two or more different health conditions at the same time
10. _____ A substantial deficit in scholastic or academic skills that is limited to a particular aspect and does not pervade all areas of learning
11. _____ An emotional response that does not fall within the traditionally accepted range of emotional reaction
12. _____ Learning disorder that includes cognitive difficulty with motor coordination, planning, and executing purposeful physical movements
13. _____ A mental health condition affecting children and teens that is characterized by a consistent pattern of aggressive and disobedient behaviors
14. _____ The development of extremely good reading skills at a very early age, ahead of word comprehension
15. _____ A disorder in the auditory cortex of the brain that disrupts how an individual's brain understands what they are hearing

A. attention-deficit/hyperactivity disorder (ADHD)
B. auditory processing disorder (APD)
C. comorbidity
D. conduct disorder
E. developmental dysphasia
F. dyscalculia
G. dysgraphia
H. dyslexia
I. dyspraxia
J. emotional dysregulation
K. executive function
L. hyperlexia
M. language processing disorder (LPD)
N. rejection sensitive dysphoria (RSD)
O. specific learning disability (SLD)

Name ______________________________ Date ______________ Class ______________

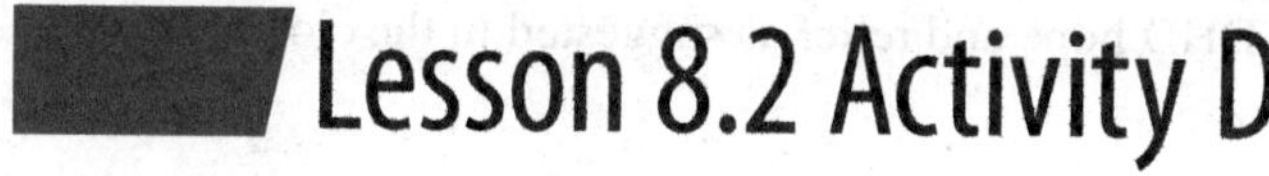

Lesson 8.2 Activity D

The Watchman Theory

Read the article below and respond to the following questions.

The Nightwatchers

The Nightwatchers sounds like something from the Marvel or DC universe! But the Watchman Theory is the premise that the ADHD brain was the perfect brain for humans during hunter-gatherer days. Specifically, consider that 70% of adults with ADHD have difficulty falling and staying asleep during periods of stress. This would have made people with ADHD the perfect nightwatchers for their clans.

The theory extends to other aspects of hunter-gatherer life as well. People with ADHD often show an ability to give equal attention to every element in their environment. Imagine how beneficial it would be for a hunter on the open plain to spot a potential bison (food source) or tiger (threat) in the corner of their field of vision? People with ADHD during these times could have been the most revered and skilled members of the clan, serving in leadership roles.

But society changed, and humans went from being nomadic hunter-gatherers roaming the land to staying in one place to farm. People worked during the day to complete chores and tasks associated with caring for the soil, plants, and animals. They minimized threats by building communities, shelters, and laws. The roots of farming societies are still present today in the industrial and technological world. Many still follow a standard workday, working patiently, quietly, and consistently. People's homes require persistent care with cleaning and yardwork.

Whereas hunter-gatherers benefited from a brain's adaptability and flexibility to tackle unknown needs and threats at a moment's notice, modern society required more patience and persistence. The ADHD brain, which would have been sought after and effective for hunter-gatherers, became less so. From the Watchman Theory's perspective, the challenge of ADHD is that people with ADHD are skilled hunter-gatherers living in a farmer's world.

For many people with ADHD, the Watchman Theory gives them hope, relief, and starts to deprogram some of the negative messages they may have received from teachers, parents, supervisors, and coworkers about their brains. It can also teach how they may be able to restructure certain aspects of their life to make it more enjoyable and be more successful.

Questions

1. How would the ADHD brain be well-suited for humans during our prehistoric past?

____

____

____

____

____

____

(Continued)

2. How could the Watchman Theory provide people with ADHD hope and relief as suggested in the closing paragraph?

3. Based on this story and the text, what strategies might you suggest that could help a person with ADHD leverage their strengths and manage the challenges of living and working in modern society?

Name ______________________________ Date ______________ Class ______________

Lesson 8.3 Activity E

Key Terms Review

Answer the following questions to review the lesson's key terms.

1. What are extensions to a diagnosis that further clarify the severity or special features of a client's disorder or illness?

____

2. What uses evidence-based techniques to teach children new skills and help them apply those skills to multiple situations through a reward-based motivation system?

____

3. What involves observing a child grow and comparing their development to typical developmental milestones?

____

4. What is the automatic repetition of words and phrases said by another person?

____

5. What provides a framework for removing barriers and providing support to address the underlying reasons for problematic behaviors?

____

6. What is the international scientific research project that aimed to map out all of the genetic information in DNA which creates the instructions for human life?

____

7. What treatment allows the child to take the lead during play while the caregivers and therapists direct the child to engage in increasingly complex interactions?

____

8. What is defined as persistent deficits across multiple environments and situations in social-emotional reciprocity, nonverbal communication used for social interaction, and developing relationships?

____

9. What is the result of a formal, in-depth developmental evaluation conducted by a trained specialist?

____

10. What refers to someone's ability to engage in social interactions between two or more people?

____

11. What is a more formal analysis of how a child is developing?

____

12. What are equipment or systems designed to maintain or improve the functional capabilities of individuals with disabilities?

____

Name ______________________ Date ______________ Class ______________

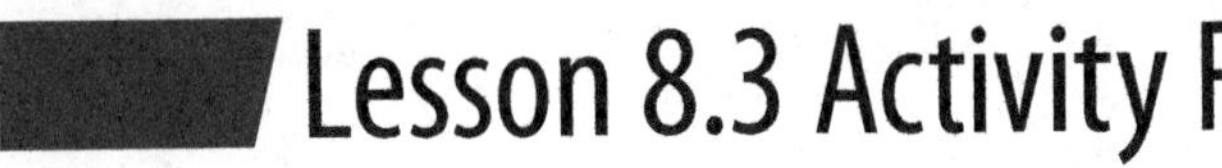

Lesson 8.3 Activity F

Reading and Understanding Data

Answer the following questions based on the information provided.

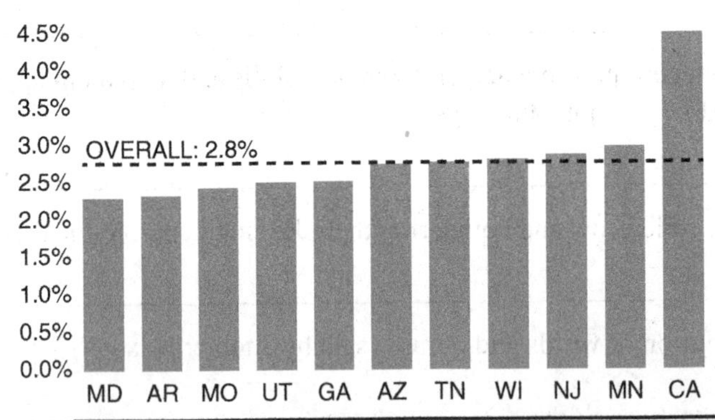

Goodheart-Willcox Publisher

1. From Figure 1, identify the three states with the highest level of children identified with autism spectrum disorder (ASD).

____

2. Which three states are the closest to the average of 2.8%?

____

For every girl identified with ASD,
boys were nearly 4 times as likely to be identified.

Goodheart-Willcox Publisher

3. Based on Figure 2, if an area has 16 girls identified with ASD, what is the expected number of boys for that area with ASD? Explain your answer.

____

____

(Continued)

Name ____

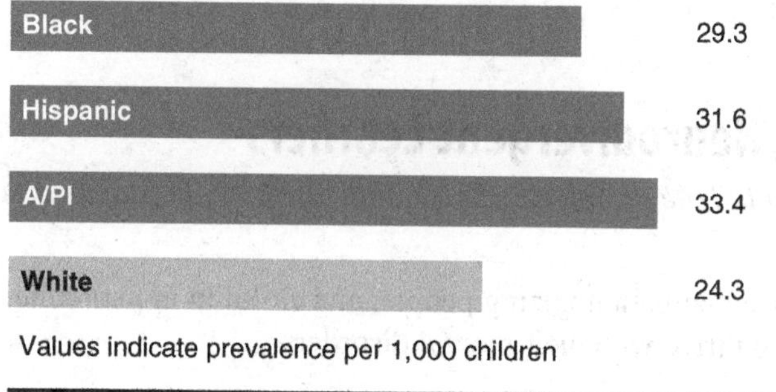

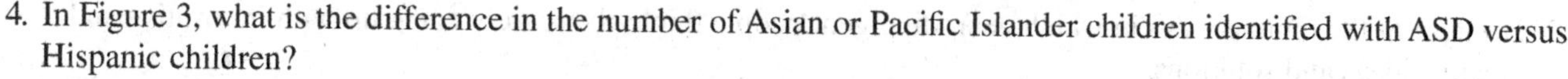

Goodheart-Willcox Publisher

4. In Figure 3, what is the difference in the number of Asian or Pacific Islander children identified with ASD versus Hispanic children?

____

5. Which two racial and ethnic groups had the lowest identification rates of ASD?

____

6. Several children identified with ASD also had an intellectual disability. The rates from this study show that one third of 8-year-old children with ASD also had an intellectual disability. At that rate, if 1,928,682 children were diagnosed with ASD, how many of these children would also have an intellectual disability?

____

Name ______________________ Date ____________ Class ____________

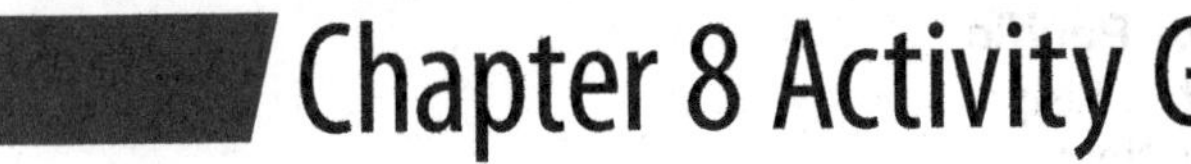

Chapter 8 Activity G

Chapter Review

Lesson 8.1 Supporting Neurodivergent Learners

For each statement, indicate if it is True or False. If False, indicate how the statement can be corrected to make it True.

1. Professional helpers recognize that pathologizing people, and children in particular, may be counterproductive to helping them learn to live and thrive with their mental disorders.

   ____

2. Because of the unique ways in which neurodivergent people think, they rarely come up with innovative and creative ideas and solutions.

   ____

3. Disability advocates encourage framing disabled people as "inspirational."

   ____

4. The goal of special education is to ensure that students with special needs have equitable access to education, receive appropriate services, and have the opportunity to reach their full potential.

   ____

5. A separate school or self-contained classroom is *never* the least restrictive environment.

   ____

6. Modifications are changes to the way the student is taught or assessed, participates in class, or completes assignments.

   ____

7. Barriers to learning exist in the environment, not in the person with the disability.

   ____

8. By making variability the rule in teaching, not the exception, more people will be able to learn information.

   ____

9. Accessibility is reactive and not proactive.

   ____

(Continued)

Name ______________________________

Lesson 8.2 Specific Learning Disabilities and ADHD

Answer the following questions.

1. _____ Specific learning disability categories include all of the following, *except* _____.
   A. attention-deficit/hyperactivity disorder
   B. developmental dysphasia
   C. executive function disorder
   D. perceptual disabilities

2. _____ Dyslexia is an example of which category of specific learning disorders?
   A. Attention-deficit/hyperactivity disorder
   B. Auditory processing disorder
   C. Conduct disorder
   D. Visual and spatial

3. _____ Which *best* characterizes nonverbal learning disorder?
   A. Cognitive difficulty with visual-spatial information, such as facial expressions, body language, drawing, or writing
   B. Challenges with planning and executing sequences of movements, such as tying shoelaces or brushing teeth
   C. Trouble with fine motor skills, such as gripping a pen or manipulating objects
   D. Struggles with number recognition, counting, and basic calculations

4. _____ Which is *not* a challenge for a person with language processing disorder?
   A. Using words correctly
   B. Handwriting
   C. Participating in group work
   D. Understanding directions

5. _____ All of the following disorders are frequent comorbidities with specific learning disabilities, *except* _____.
   A. anxiety disorders
   B. conduct disorder
   C. depressive disorders
   D. personality disorders

6. _____ ADHD is characterized with difficulty paying attention, controlling impulsive behaviors, or _____.
   A. aggressiveness
   B. being overly active
   C. coordinating motor functions
   D. interpreting visual information

7. _____ Which *best* characterizes people ADHD's experience?
   A. Difficulty regulating or shifting attention
   B. Little impact on home, work, or school life
   C. Inability to focus
   D. Highly organized and orderly

8. _____ Low levels of which two neurotransmitters are linked to ADHD?
   A. Serotonin and gamma-aminobutyric acid
   B. Gamma-aminobutyric acid and norepinephrine
   C. Norepinephrine and dopamine
   D. Dopamine and serotonin

9. _____ Which is *least likely* a sign of ADHD?
   A. Trouble sitting still
   B. Using words incorrectly
   C. Making careless mistakes
   D. Interrupting or blurting out answers

(Continued)

10. _____ Which comorbid disorder is a person with ADHD *most likely* to experience?
A. Memory disorder
B. Personality disorder
C. Rejection sensitive dysphoria
D. Schizophrenia spectrum disorder

Lesson 8.3 Autism Spectrum Disorder

Fill in the blank to answer the following questions.

1. Eventually, autism came to be viewed as its own developmental disorder with its own set of criteria, including a lack of interest in people, atypical responses to the environment, and severe impairments in _____.

____

2. In the 1990s, three disorders emerged under the umbrella of autism, which included childhood disintegrative disorder, Rett syndrome, and _____.

____

3. By 2013, _____ emerged as the formal diagnosis of a range of symptoms in part in response to concerns around inconsistent diagnosis.

____

Classify the following ASD behavior examples into one of three clusters: social communication and interaction (A), restrictive or repetitive behaviors or interests (B), or other characteristics (C).

4. _____ Flaps hands, rocks body, or spins self in circles
5. _____ Does not notice when others are hurt or upset by 24 months of age
6. _____ Gastrointestinal issues (for example, constipation)
7. _____ Sensory difficulties including hypersensitive or hyposensitive
8. _____ Gets upset by minor changes
9. _____ Does not show facial expressions like happy, sad, angry, and surprised by 9 months of age
10. _____ Lack of fear or more fear than expected
11. _____ Avoids or does not keep eye contact
12. _____ Has obsessive interests

For each item below, indicate if the statement is True or False. If False, indicate how to correct the statement to make it True.

13. The goal of ASD treatment is to maximize the person's ability to function by reducing symptoms and supporting development, learning, and functioning.

____

14. ASD treatment may require the coordination of a team of professionals from a variety of specialties to meet the specific needs of a child, known as an inter-agency collaborative team.

____

15. Applied behavior analysis (ABA) lets the child take the lead during play, while the caregivers and therapists direct the child to engage in increasingly complex interactions.

____

Name ______________________ Date ____________ Class ____________

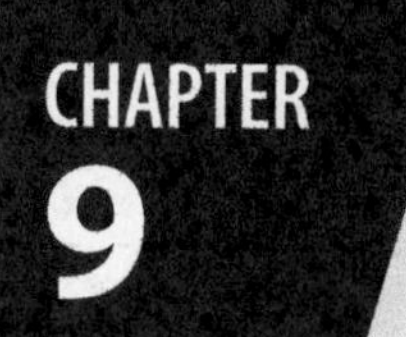

Mental Disorder

Lesson 9.1 Activity A

Rosenhan's Pseudopatients

In 1975, American psychologist David Rosenhan published a paper called "On Being Sane in Insane Places." The paper outlined his research on mental institutions. The following summarizes this two-phase study.

Phase 1

- Eight undercover pseudopatients, or fake patients, who were mentally well (not hearing voices), checked into a mental institution reporting that they had been hearing voices.
- After being admitted, the pseudopatients stopped presenting their fake symptoms and behaved normally, waiting to be recognized as mentally healthy.
- The fake patients were forced to take medications, which they spit out.
- They were kept for an average of 19 days, with one being kept for 52 days.
- Upon discharge, they received a diagnosis of "paranoid schizophrenia, in remission" (which is no longer a diagnosis in the DSM).

Phase 2

- Rosenhan shared his findings with a teaching hospital, telling staff that he would be sending more pseudopatients, challenging them to detect the fake patients.
- Of 193 new patients, the staff identified 41 as likely or suspected pseudopatients.
- Rosenhan never sent any fake patients.

In his 1975 paper, Rosenhan argued that mental health diagnoses should be viewed as a curable or treatable illness, rather than an irreversible condition. While some mental illnesses are chronic, Rosenhan argued that diagnosing a patient with a disorder flagged "in remission" permanently labeled them as mentally ill. He also found that reporting something very atypical, such as hearing voices in your head once, is much more alarming to a provider than weeks of normal behavior.

Rosenhan's experiment and findings were criticized. One criticism was that the study only showed that it was possible to deceive clinicians by lying to them. However, the paper was successful in sparking important debates among those in the field of counseling and mental health. How should mental disorders be defined, diagnosed, and classified? What should mental health treatment look like? How could a mental disorder diagnosis negatively affect people?

1. Imagine yourself as one of Rosenhan's pseudopatients. Describe the emotions you may have experienced over the course of your time in a 1970s psychiatric hospital.

____

____

____

____

(Continued)

2. Why do you think "in remission" is no longer a diagnosis in the DSM?

3. In phase two of the study, what percentage of new patients did the psychiatric hospital staff identify as likely or suspected pseudopatients?

4. In phase two of the study, why is it significant that the staff identified 41 new patients as likely or suspected pseudopatients?

5. A criticism of the research methodology of Rosenhan's study is the small sample size. It provides a snapshot of one psychiatric hospital, in one geographical area, at one moment in time. Therefore, many caution applying these findings to modern mental health diagnosis and treatment. What has changed in mental health diagnosis and treatment since the 1970s that may make the findings less relevant?

6. Rosenhan's study coincided with the deinstitutionalization movement (as covered in Lesson 1.1). What do you think the findings of his study had on this movement?

Name ______________________ Date ______________ Class ______________

Lesson 9.1 Activity B

Key Terms Review

Fill in the blanks in the following statements to review the lesson's key terms.

1. In the context of the patterns of thinking or feeling in a mental disorder, _____ means spread through an individual, impacting cognition, emotion, and behavior.

   ____

2. _____ is the negative social view of a characteristic of an individual as a mental, physical, or social deficiency.

   ____

3. Classifying a person according to a mental disorder criteria and characteristics of those criteria is called _____.

   ____

4. A disorder that is causing a deviation from what would be considered typical is called _____.

   ____

5. A belief or expectation that helps to bring about its own fulfillment is called _____.

   ____

6. The term _____ is used when a person is showing signs of distress, deviance, and dysfunction, but they do not have the full number of symptoms to meet the formal diagnosis.

   ____

7. _____ means that the disorder is causing stress or harm to the person and/or the people around them.

   ____

8. _____ is a sociological hypothesis that if a person is described in terms of particular behavioral characteristics, it may have a significant effect on their behavior.

   ____

9. Behaviors that sharply deviate from social norms and violate other people's rights are called _____.

   ____

10. Discrimination against people with mental or physical disabilities is called _____.

    ____

11. _____ means that the disorder is making it difficult for the person to function in society.

    ____

12. The _____ is the handbook used by experts and professionals in the United States, and much of the world, as the authoritative guide to the diagnosis of mental disorders.

    ____

13. _____ is mostly used in a situation where the clinician does not have enough time to determine the client's specific disorder, but it is clear that they are in need of services within the family of conditions.

    ____

Name ______________________ Date ______________ Class ____________

Lesson 9.2 Activity C

Key Terms Review

Review the lesson's key terms by matching the term with the example.

1. _____ Persistent irrational fears of specific objects, activities, or situations
2. _____ Disorder characterized by anxiety related to interacting or being seen by others
3. _____ Disorder characterized by continued tension and apprehension
4. _____ Subset of major depressive disorder that is qualified with a seasonal pattern of depressive symptoms
5. _____ Disorder characterized by prolonged hopelessness and lethargy
6. _____ Disorders characterized by distressful, persistent anxiety and the maladaptive behaviors that reduce that anxiety
7. _____ A mood disorder where a person alternates between the hopelessness and lethargy of depression and the over-excited state of mania
8. _____ Episodes of intense dread or fear that come suddenly and without warning
9. _____ Irrational thoughts that shape how you see the world, feel, and act
10. _____ Disorder characterized by recurring intrusive thoughts that prompt the performance of neutralizing rituals
11. _____ A hyperactive, wildly optimistic emotional state that is characteristic of a mood disorder
12. _____ An emotion characterized by worry and bodily symptoms of tension in which an individual anticipates impending danger, catastrophe, or misfortune
13. _____ Disorder characterized by a prolonged, pervasive emotional disturbance
14. _____ Mental events that interrupt the flow of task-related thoughts despite efforts to avoid them

A. anxiety
B. anxiety disorders
C. bipolar disorder
D. cognitive distortion
E. generalized anxiety disorder (GAD)
F. intrusive thoughts
G. major depressive disorder
H. mania
I. mood disorder
J. obsessive-compulsive disorder (OCD)
K. panic attacks
L. phobias
M. seasonal affective disorder
N. social anxiety disorder

Name ______________________ Date ______________ Class ______________

Lesson 9.2 Activity D

Recognizing Symptoms

For each scenario, indicate if the person is most likely experiencing an anxiety disorder, an obsessive-compulsive disorder, a mood disorder, or if there is not enough information. If a specific disorder or subcategory is present, indicate the specific disorder or subcategory.

1. On his way to work, Pluto wonders if he turned off the oven after making breakfast. He calls his partner who works from home to double-check that the oven is off.

   ____

   ____

2. Jasmine has a fear of crowds that prevents her from going out with her friends to festivals or clubs and has kept her from accepting a promotion at work because it would involve attending large conferences.

   ____

   ____

3. Sonja's attention is fixated on her weight. It takes her hours to get ready for work in the morning, with most of that time spent looking at herself in the mirror. She tries on outfit after outfit to find the clothes that hide her body shape the best. On the weekends, she cancels plans with her friends because she's afraid of being judged by others.

   ____

   ____

4. Eric has been feeling constantly tense or "on edge" that something bad is going to happen soon. This feeling has resulted in him feeling powerless, stuck, and losing sleep. He can't identify a specific thing that has him worried. By moment, it could be politics, the environment, what others think about him, or what others may be saying about him.

   ____

   ____

5. For the last month, Hui has been feeling down. He's only doing the things he has to do, like show up for work. Instead of taking care of housework, exercising, or spending time with friends, he feels an intense need to just lay in bed. He thinks about getting up, but it's as if there is a heavy blanket holding him down that he can't remove. He's starting to wonder why he even exists.

   ____

   ____

6. A few weeks ago, Maria was laid off from work. Since then, she has been feeling down and discouraged. She sent out some résumés and talked to a couple former colleagues who made some introductions for her with potential new employers. She is feeling discouraged, resentful, and anxious about her prospects for finding a new job.

   ____

   ____

(Continued)

7. Since Tuesday, Alejandro has been more energetic than usual at the coffee shop where he works. He runs around, knocks out orders at twice the speed, and is overly outgoing with customers. Each night, he's pressured by at least one friend to go out, staying up until 2:00 a.m. despite needing to be at work at 6:30 a.m. But when he woke up on Saturday, he felt a lot of guilt, wouldn't text any of his friends or family back, and his speech was noticeably slower than the last few days.

____

____

8. Morgan is hanging out with his partner on the beach when, suddenly and without warning, a pain shoots through his chest, his heartbeat starts racing, and he struggles to breathe. He is filled with an overwhelming sense of dread. His partner recognizes what is going on. Remaining calm, Morgan's partner asks him to name five things he sees, four he can touch, three he hears, two he can smell, and one he can taste. Slowly, Morgan's breathing becomes easier, his heart rate slows, and the feeling of dread subsides.

____

____

9. Solidad's apartment is littered with old shipping boxes and bags and used food containers that she cannot throw away. Even though she is embarrassed to have people over and struggles to move around and use her living space, she cannot throw these items out because she believes she may need them and won't have them.

____

____

10. Martha recently gave birth to her first child. But unlike what she thought would happen, she is filled with intense feelings of sadness and indifference to her child. She has no appetite and is sleeping a lot more than usual. She's feeling a lot of shame and guilt about her behavior and emotions. After all, this period is supposed to be filled with warmth, love, and bonding with her new child. Her partner is also concerned and helps her make an appointment to see her doctor.

____

____

Name ______________________ Date ____________ Class ____________

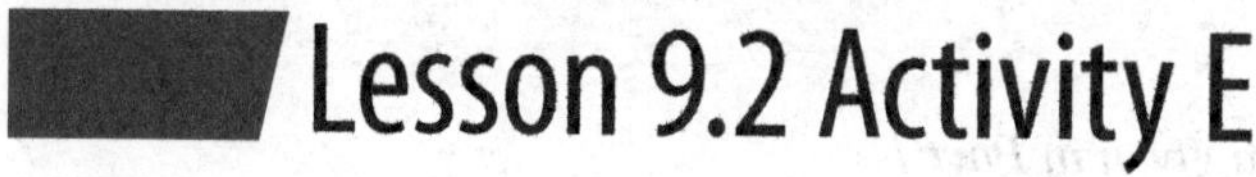

Lesson 9.2 Activity E

Statistics of Disorders

Review the facts and statistics about anxiety disorders. Answer the questions about the facts below.

Part 1

Generalized Anxiety Disorder (GAD)

- GAD affects 6.8 million adults or 3.1% of the U.S. population, yet only 43.2% are receiving treatment. NIMH: Generalized Anxiety Disorder.
- Women are twice as likely to be affected as men. GAD often co-occurs with major depression.

Panic Disorder (PD)

- PD affects 6 million adults or 2.7% of the U.S. population. NIMH: Panic Disorders.
- Women are twice as likely to be affected as men.

Social Anxiety Disorder

- SAD affects 15 million adults or 7.1% of the U.S. population. NIMH: Social Anxiety Disorder.
- SAD is equally common among men and women and typically begins around age 13.

Specific Phobias

- Specific phobias affect 19.3 million adults or 9.1% of the U.S. population. NIMH: Specific Phobias.
- Women are twice as likely to be affected as men.
- Symptoms typically begin in childhood; the average age of onset is 7 years old.

Obsessive-Compulsive Disorder (OCD)

- OCD affects 2.5 million adults or 1.2% of the U.S. population. NIMH: Obsessive-Compulsive Disorder.
- Women are 3x more likely to be affected as men.
- The average age of onset is 19, with 25% of cases occurring by age 14. One-third of affected adults first experienced symptoms in childhood.

1. Which disorder impacts the most people in the United States?

   ____

2. Women are impacted at a higher rate than men in many of the disorders. Which disorders impact women at rates two times higher than men?

   ____

3. Which disorder impacts women at a rate even higher than two times more than the rate it impacts men?

   ____

4. What disorder is equally present between men and women?

   ____

5. At what age do social anxiety symptoms often start?

   ____

(Continued)

Part 2

Identify the correct disorders in the graph, based on the data given in Part 1.

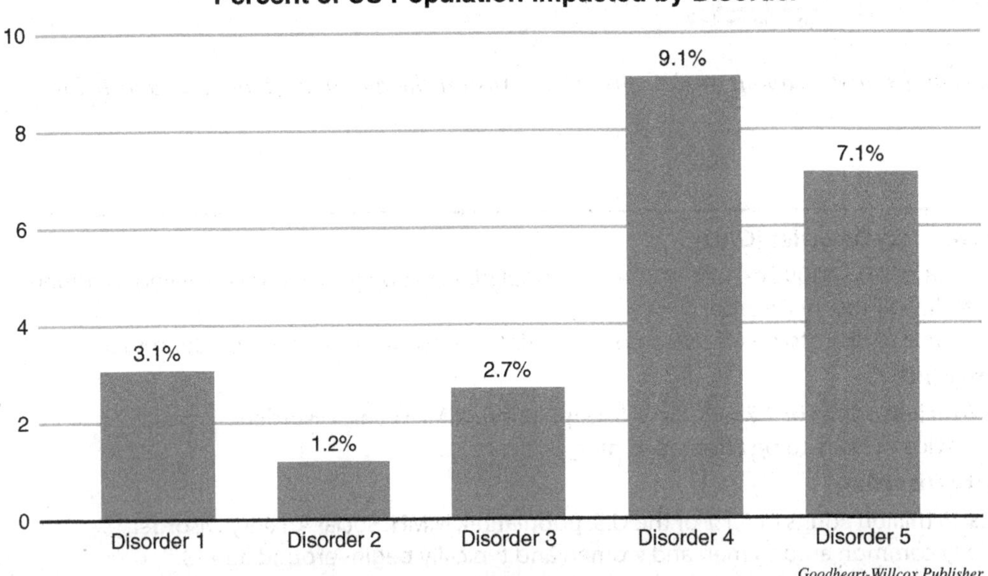

Goodheart-Willcox Publisher

1. What is Disorder 1?

____

2. What is Disorder 2?

____

3. What is Disorder 3?

____

4. What is Disorder 4?

____

5. What is Disorder 5?

____

Name ______________________ Date ____________ Class ____________

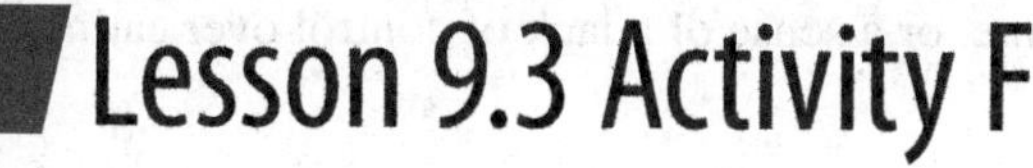

Lesson 9.3 Activity F

Key Terms Review

Part 1

Answer the following questions to review the lesson's key terms.

1. When a behavior is characterized by abnormal movements, behaviors, and withdrawal, it is described as what?

   ____

2. What is the theory that mental and physical disorders develop from a genetic or biological predisposition for that disorder combined with stressful conditions?

   ____

3. What is an eating disorder characterized by persistent restriction of energy intake relative to the person; intense fear of gaining weight or becoming fat; and distorted body image?

   ____

4. What are deficits in the ability to perform normal functions of living that present as apathy, inability to express emotions through body language and tone, emotional withdrawal, poor rapport, and lack of spontaneity?

   ____

5. A group of disorders characterized by disruption in the normal integration of consciousness, memory, or perception of the environment is called what?

   ____

6. What is a disorder characterized by a lack of conscience for wrongdoing even toward family and friends?

   ____

7. What is a psychotic disorder characterized by disturbances in thinking, emotional responsiveness, and behavior?

   ____

8. What is a disorder characterized by recurring episodes of binge eating followed by compensatory behaviors to prevent weight gain?

   ____

9. What is an eating disorder characterized by binge-eating episodes associated with three or more of the following: eating more rapidly than normal, eating until uncomfortably full, eating large amounts when not hungry, and/or eating alone out of embarrassment?

   ____

10. What describes when the impulses, thoughts, or behaviors of a person are distressful to one's sense of self?

    ____

11. What is an eating disorder characterized by a disturbance in eating resulting in persistent failure to meet nutritional needs and extreme picky eating?

    ____

(Continued)

12. Eating more than most people would eat in a period of time, or a sense of a lack of control over eating, is called what?

____

13. What disorders involve pervasive and recurring patterns of perceiving, relating to, and thinking about the environment and the self that interfere with long-term functioning?

____

14. What means that the impulses, thoughts, or behaviors of the person experiencing them are compatible with their sense of self?

____

15. A cluster of disorders involving a pathological disturbance of attitudes, behaviors, and emotions related to food is called what?

____

Part 2

Match the disorder with the symptoms.

1. _____ A person blocks out specific information
2. _____ A person experiences a feeling of being alienated from others and society as a whole
3. _____ A person may travel for months with no awareness of their identity
4. _____ A person experiences a feeling that their extremities have changed in size
5. _____ A person has no memory of a particular event
6. _____ A person exhibits more than one distinct personality

A. Dissociative amnesia
B. Dissociative fugue
C. Dissociative identity disorder
D. Depersonalization disorder

Name ______________________ Date ____________ Class ____________

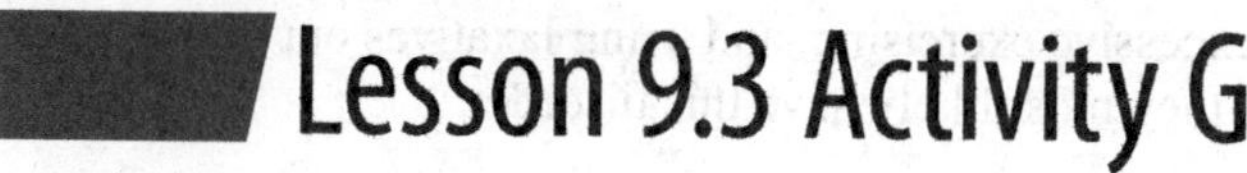

Lesson 9.3 Activity G

Disorder Jeopardy

Match the disorder listed below with the symptom or trait listed.

Anorexia nervosa	Dissociative fugue
Antisocial personality disorder	Dissociative identity disorder
Avoidant personality disorder	Histrionic personality disorder
Avoidant-restrictive food intake disorder	Narcissistic personality disorder
Binge-eating disorder	Obsessive-compulsive personality disorder
Borderline personality disorder	Paranoid personality disorder
Bulimia nervosa	Schizoid personality disorder
Dependent personality disorder	Schizotypal personality disorder
Depersonalization disorder	Schizophrenia spectrum disorder
Dissociative amnesia	

1. With this disorder, a person exhibits grandiose self-importance, exaggerated sense of talent and achievements, a need for admiration, and a lack of empathy.

   ____

2. This disorder is characterized by an inability to recall a memory or specific information of an event.

   ____

3. This disorder is characterized by intense feelings of depression, guilt, and shame following episodes of eating more than most people would in a period of time without any compensatory behavior.

   ____

4. If a person demonstrates emotional coldness, no tenderness for others, lack of a desire for close relationships, and an indifference to praise or criticism and the feelings of others, they most likely have this disorder.

   ____

5. Most well-known for the symptom of hallucinations, this disorder typically emerges between late adolescents to the mid-30s.

   ____

6. Often associated with the words "psychopath" or "sociopath," this disorder is largely characterized by a disposition to disregard and violate the rights of others.

   ____

7. If a person exhibits hypersensitivity to rejection and criticism, a desire for uncritical acceptance, social withdrawal in spite of a desire for affection and acceptance, and low self-esteem, they most likely have this disorder.

   ____

8. With this disorder, a person has an extreme need for perfection, is excessively orderly, cannot compromise, and has an exaggerated sense of moral responsibility.

   ____

(Continued)

9. If a person exhibits signs of extreme calorie restriction, excessive exercising, and using laxatives out of an intense fear of gaining weight or a distorted body image, they most likely have this disorder.

____

10. With this disorder, a person's mood, interpersonal relationships, and self-image is highly unstable to the point that it is affecting their ability to function socially and in their career.

____

11. This disorder can be experienced as a feeling that the world is not real, like they are an avatar in a game simulation, and self-estrangement.

____

12. With this disorder, a person has episodes of eating more than most would in a period of time and then using a compensatory behavior like vomiting or fasting to prevent weight gain, which is important since their self-worth is highly dependent on their body image.

____

13. A person who is exhibiting unwarranted suspicion and distrust, is easily offended, is always ready to strike back, and restricts affection toward others most likely has this disorder.

____

14. This disorder is believed to be associated with severe physical or sexual abuse, is highly debated among professionals, and is characterized by the presentation of more than one distinct personality in a person.

____

15. The symptoms of this disorder do not warrant a schizophrenia diagnosis, but the person displays similar symptoms like peculiar thoughts, perceptions, speech, and behavior.

____

Name ______________________________ Date ______________ Class ______________

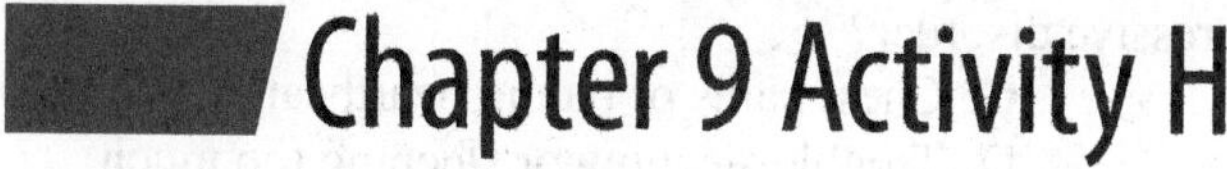

Chapter 9 Activity H

Chapter Review

Lesson 9.1 Diagnosis

Based on the information provided, indicate "Disorder" if the person is most likely dealing with a mental disorder or "No Disorder" if the person is displaying typical behavior or experiencing mental distress.

1. Andy is unable to maintain employment.

   ____

2. Nene is depressed after being laid off of work.

   ____

3. Caroline has set a goal to be more physically fit so she exercises 4 days a week and tries to increase her protein intake in her diet.

   ____

4. Terry has no real friends and several estranged relatives.

   ____

5. Most days, Vicki exercises two to three times a day, often declining invitations to spend time with friends and family to exercise, and she stops eating for the day after consuming 1,000 calories.

   ____

For each statement below, fill in the blank.

6. _____ may provide an incomplete or misleading representation of a person's condition and situation.

   ____

7. Stigma can lead to _____, or discrimination against people with mental or physical disabilities.

   ____

Lesson 9.2 Anxiety, Obsessive-Compulsive, and Mood Disorders

Answer the following questions.

1. _____ Unlike phobias, which have a specific perceived threat, people with generalized anxiety disorder (GAD) _____.
   - A. have sudden onset episodes of intense anxiety that can feel like a heart attack
   - B. are distressed by intrusive thoughts that compel them to perform neutralizing rituals
   - C. experience near-constant anxiety that can shift between a wide range of concerns
   - D. feel anxious when interacting with or being around others, like at parties, restaurants, conferences, or festivals

2. _____ Which *best* describes the experience of someone with obsessive-compulsive disorder?
   - A. They feel intense, unbearable anxiety about intrusive thoughts.
   - B. They experience emotional extremes and challenges in regulating mood.
   - C. They become obsessed with a perceived flaw in their physical appearance.
   - D. They cannot overcome the compulsion to pull hair out of their scalp or eyebrows.

(Continued)

3. _____ Which symptom is *not* associated with a major depressive disorder?
A. Thoughts of death or suicide
B. Slowed movements or speech
C. Chest pains or racing heartbeat
D. Trouble sleeping or sleeping too much

4. _____ All of the following are symptoms of mania *except* _____.
A. delusions of grandeur
B. feeling worthless or guilty
C. engaging in risky behavior
D. high, uncontrollable energy

5. _____ The social cognitive perspective suggests that people who suffer from mood disorders adopt a negative lens. One contributing factor may be when people believe they lack control over events in their environment, which results in a lack of motivation to make changes or try to impact change. What does this describe?
A. Self-blame
B. "Should" thoughts
C. Emotional reasoning
D. Learned helplessness

6. _____ All of the following are symptoms of overthinking *except* _____.
A. difficulty making decisions and second-guessing decisions
B. assuming that something is true based on your emotional response to it
C. needing others to provide reassurance or validate your thoughts, feelings, or behaviors
D. overly replaying an experience in your mind or imagining how you will handle future situations

Lesson 9.3 Other Disorders

For each statement below, indicate if the statement is True or False. If False, indicate how to correct the statement to make it True.

1. The diathesis-stress model explains why some people with a genetic predisposition may never develop schizophrenia and why rates tend to be higher among people who experience poverty or socioeconomic stress.

____

2. The catatonic behavior associated with schizophrenia may present as apathy, inability to express emotions through body language and tone, emotional withdrawal, poor rapport, or a lack of spontaneity.

____

3. Dissociative amnesia is characterized by a person suddenly setting out on a journey for hours or months and traveling around with no awareness of their identity.

____

Answer the following questions.

4. _____ Eating disorders are _____.
A. mental disorders that affect women
B. physiological disorders and not mental disorders
C. solely the result of physiological and genetic factors
D. serious mental disorders that can even cause death, but they are treatable

5. _____ All of the following are sociocultural factors contributing to eating disorders *except* which one?
A. Valuing thinness as morally virtuous
B. Individual and family history of mental disorders
C. Over-emphasizing weight when evaluating health
D. Viewing individual decisions as the sole factor of a person's weight

6. _____ Which *best* outlines an individual, psychological factor that contributes to eating disorders?
A. Increased pressure for girls and women to have a certain body size or shape
B. Indicators like the BMI and media representations that reflect white, European standards of attractiveness and health
C. A need for control, anxiety about gaining weight, and feelings of worthlessness and hopelessness
D. Public opinions around healthy diet and exercise that largely focus on foods, products, and fitness programs that are more expensive

Name ______________________ Date ______________ Class ______________

CHAPTER 10

Treatment

Lesson 10.1 Activity A

Cognitive Distortions

For each type of cognitive distortion, provide an example different from those covered in the text.

Cognitive Distortion	Example
Dichotomous thinking	
Overgeneralization	
Selective abstraction	
Disqualifying the positive	
Mind reading	
Fortune telling	
Minimization	
Catastrophizing	
Emotional reasoning	
"Should" statements	
Attribution (personalization)	
Attribution (blame)	

Name ______________________ Date ____________ Class ____________

Lesson 10.1 Activity B

Key Terms Review

Fill in the blanks in the following statements to review the lesson's key terms.

1. _____ is a modality that emphasizes changing maladaptive behaviors.

   ____

2. Any psychological service provided by a trained professional that primarily uses forms of communication and interaction is called _____.

   ____

3. A modality based on the principle that emotional and behavioral problems are the result of maladaptive or faulty ways of thinking and distorted attitudes about oneself and others is called _____.

   ____

4. _____ are underlying, long-term beliefs a person has that help them understand how the world works and who they are.

   ____

5. _____ are therapeutic and counseling techniques or processes.

   ____

6. _____ is one of the most widely used modalities, which includes a variety of techniques that use the interrelationships between thoughts, behaviors, and feelings.

   ____

7. _____ occurs when a person develops thought or behavior patterns that are harmful to, are counterproductive to, or otherwise interfere with optimal functioning in various domains of life.

   ____

8. In _____, a therapist introduces an effective interpersonal skill that the client practices until they are ready to apply the skill in the real world.

   ____

9. _____ is when a therapist pairs training in deep muscle relaxation with the presentation of anxiety-provoking situations for the client.

   ____

10. _____ is the process of identifying cognitive distortions and replacing them with more adaptive cognitions.

    ____

11. _____ is the use of a device to provide a client with information about their physiological state and then providing training to teach that person how to voluntarily control body functions like heart rate.

    ____

12. _____ are a person's instant, unconscious interpretations of events.

    ____

13. Assumptions, attitudes, and rules that people apply to a variety of situations are called _____.

    ____

Name ______________________ Date ____________ Class ____________

Lesson 10.2 Activity C

Key Terms Review

Review the lesson's key terms by matching the term with the example.

1. _____ An approach to treatment that involves selecting techniques from different therapeutic modalities that best meet the needs of the client
2. _____ Type of therapy that helps the client increase their awareness and understanding of their feelings and emotions, be present, and accept responsibility for their behaviors
3. _____ Type of therapy that treats mental disorders through physical methods that directly influence the body
4. _____ A therapist's warmth, receptiveness, lack of judgment, and avoidance of coming across as an authoritative figure
5. _____ Drugs that work to influence people's mental, emotional, and behavioral processes by increasing or decreasing certain neurotransmitters in the brain
6. _____ Type of therapy that focuses more on helping the client recognize and exercise their free will, develop self-determination, and search for the meaning in events, relationships, and life
7. _____ Type of therapy in which the therapist creates a nonjudgmental space and actively listens, acknowledges, and paraphrases concerns to ensure they understand the client's experience
8. _____ An unseen but influential basic, natural force within humans, or in some views, all living things, that seeks connection with the forces of nature, humankind, the universe, and the unknown
9. _____ Therapy that involves analysis of drives and motivations while focusing on processes of change and how a client's personality is influenced by their interpersonal relationships
10. _____ The ability to notice internal sensations in the body, including heart rate, breathing, hunger or fullness, temperature, pain, and emotional sensations
11. _____ Any practice that brings great awareness and connection with the forces of nature, humankind, the universe, and the unknown
12. _____ The administration of drugs to treat mental disorders
13. _____ Therapy that adopts a more holistic approach that focuses on free will, human potential, and self-discovery
14. _____ The use of any physiological intervention to treat the psychological symptoms of mental disorders

A. biomedical therapy
B. client-centered therapy
C. existential therapy
D. Gestalt therapy
E. humanistic therapy
F. integrative therapy
G. interoceptive awareness
H. pharmacotherapy
I. psychodynamic therapy
J. psychotropic medications
K. somatic therapy
L. spirit
M. spirituality
N. unconditional positive regard

Name ______________________ Date ______________ Class ____________

Lesson 10.2 Activity D

Recognizing Modalities

Indicate which modality each statement best exemplifies.

Brainspotting	Humanistic therapy
Classical psychoanalysis	Integrative therapy
Client-centered therapy	Psychodynamic therapy
Eye-movement desensitization reprocessing	Somatic therapy
Gestalt therapy	Transcranial magnetic stimulation

1. Most clinicians use this modality, which does not see any one method as better than another, nor does it shy away from using theories that contradict each other.

   ____

2. This modality focuses heavily on a client's unconscious drives by analyzing such things as psychosexual motivations and dreams.

   ____

3. This therapy uses bilateral sensory stimulation to help clients process and heal from past trauma.

   ____

4. Breathwork is a technique used in this modality, which focuses on using the connection between mind and body to help clients.

   ____

5. An example of a therapy from this modality is existential therapy, which helps people exercise their free will and find meaning in events, relationships, and life.

   ____

6. This therapy is most often used when a client is not responding to other depression treatments, like antidepressants.

   ____

7. This modality relies heavily on unconditional positive regard and has the goal of helping the client get in touch with their true self and develop a deeper and more accurate understanding of themself.

   ____

8. This modality helps clients explore their feelings and emotions, be more present in the moment, and accept responsibility for their choices and behaviors.

   ____

9. This modality uses talk therapy to understand the relationship between motivations, personality, and the mind.

   ____

10. This technique may be used to help clients heal from traumatic events by identifying points in their field of vision where trauma is stored and having them recall the event in a safe therapeutic environment.

    ____

Name ______________________ Date ____________ Class ____________

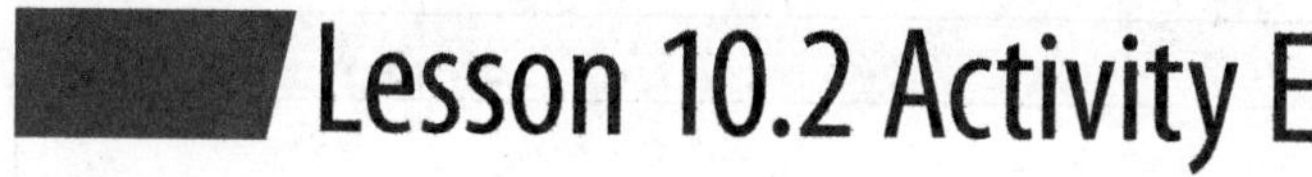

Lesson 10.2 Activity E

Psychotropic Medication Research

Identify two medications from two different classifications to research, and record your notes in the table below. Then, develop a presentation using the methods approved by your teacher.

Prompt	Response
Medication #1	
Classification	
When it is used	
How it works	
Effectiveness	
How to take it or precautions in starting or stopping	
Side effects	

(Continued)

Prompt	Response
Medication #2	
Classification	
When it is used	
How it works	
Effectiveness	
How to take it or precautions in starting or stopping	
Side effects	

Name ____________________ Date ____________ Class ____________

Lesson 10.2 Activity F

Treatment Data

Review the following charts of data gathered by the National Center for Health Statistics regarding mental health treatments. Then, answer the questions that follow.

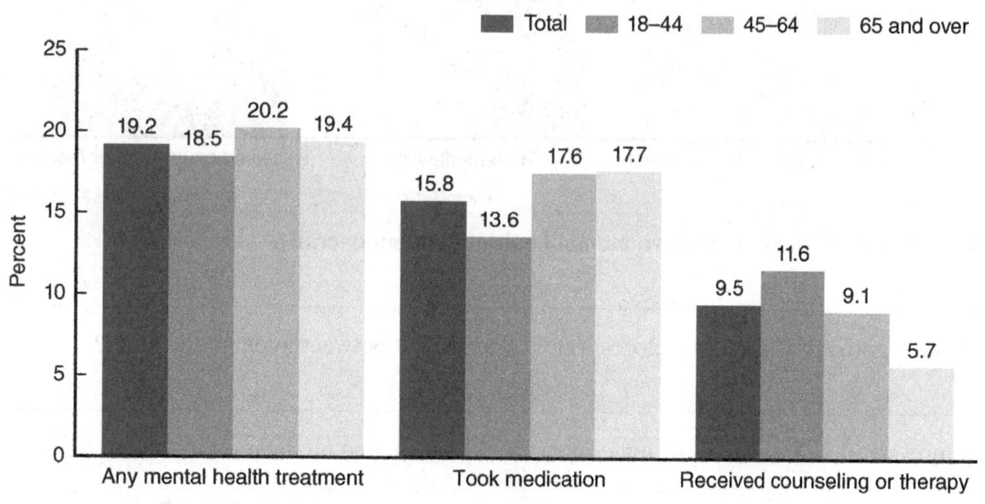

1. Which age group had the highest rate of receiving any mental health treatment?

____

2. Which age group took medication at the highest rate?

____

3. Which age group received counseling or therapy at the highest rate?

____

4. What conclusions can you draw about mental health treatment by age based on this data?

____

____

____

Note on the data: Adults were considered to have received any mental health treatment if they reported having taken medication for their mental health, received counseling or therapy from a mental health professional, or both in the past 12 months. Adults were asked separately if they took prescription medication for feelings of anxiety, for depression, or to help with any other emotions or with their concentration, behavior, or mental health. Adults who responded positively to any of these three questions were considered to have taken medication for their mental health in the past 12 months. Estimates are based on household interviews of a sample of the U.S. civilian noninstitutionalized population.

(Continued)

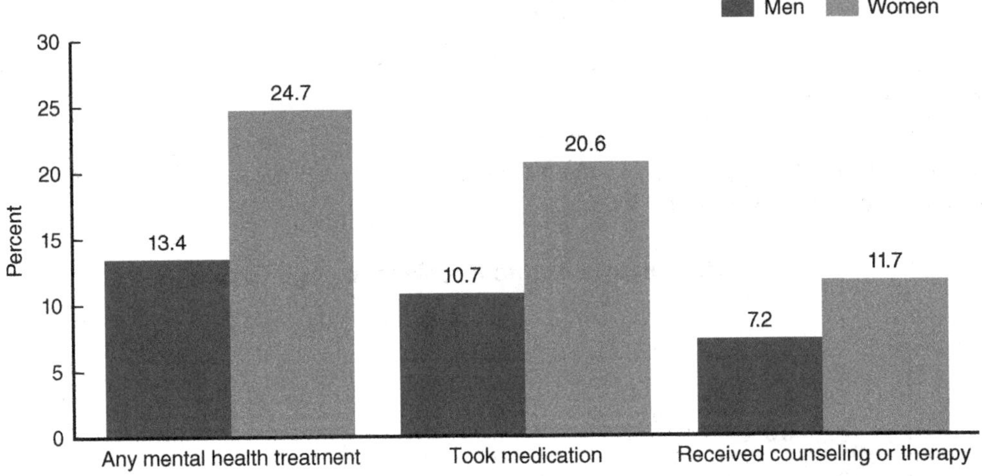

5. Are men or women more likely to receive mental health treatment overall?

6. Which treatment approach showed the closest rates of treatment between men and women?

7. If this data represented 1,000 men, how many men would have taken medication in the last year?

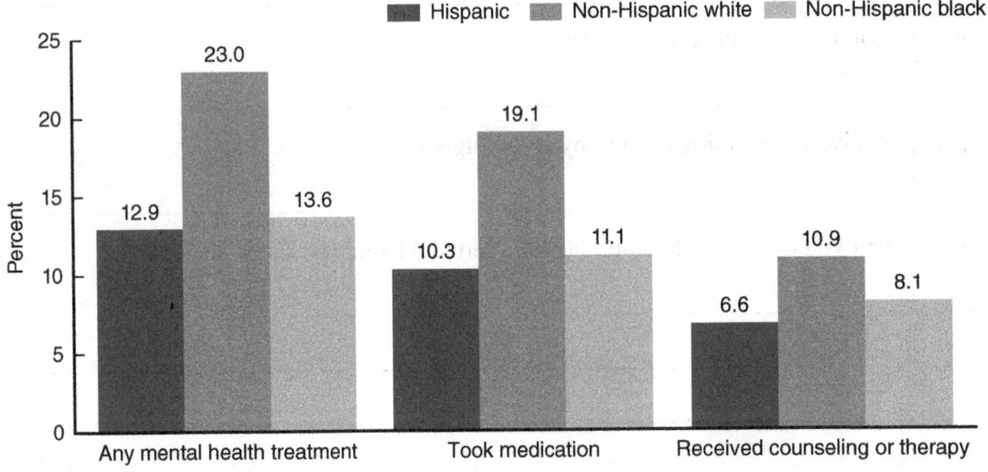

8. Which group had the highest rate of receiving any mental health treatment?

9. What treatment approach showed the closest rates of treatment between the group with the highest rates and the group with the lowest rates?

10. What was the difference between the rate at which Non-Hispanic white adults took medication and the rate at which Hispanic adults took medication?

Name ______________________ Date ____________ Class ____________

Lesson 10.3 Activity G

Key Terms Review

Answer the following questions to review the lesson's key terms.

1. When the counselor provides less formal guidance and advice on issues between partners, this is called what?

   ____

2. What is the application of treatment modalities on a one-on-one basis?

   ____

3. What is a treatment for mental disorders in which multiple participants interact with each other on an emotional and cognitive level, along with one or more helpers who serve as facilitators?

   ____

4. What are areas in which the counselor has specific knowledge, certification, or experience?

   ____

5. What involves providing specialized instruction and training to enable individuals to acquire or enhance particular skills or improve performance?

   ____

6. What type of therapy focuses on improving relationships within the family and behavior patterns of the family unit as a whole, as well as among individual members and groupings within the family?

   ____

7. When both partners in a committed relationship are treated at the same time by the same therapist or therapists, this is called what?

   ____

8. What is a form of family therapy in which the infant or young child and caregiver are treated together?

   ____

Name ______________________ Date ____________ Class ____________

Lesson 10.3 Activity H

Reflecting on a Specialty

Select a specialty in counseling and mental health that interests you. Figure 10.13 provides some examples of specialties, but there are others you may choose as well. You can research specialties that counselors and therapists list on their online profiles.
Then, use the space below to write a reflection using one of the following prompts.

- "I'm interested in this speciality because…"
- "This speciality is important because…"
- "This therapy involves…"
- "This group has unique needs such as…"

1. What is your selected specialty?

____

2. Chosen prompt:

____

3. Reflection from prompt:

____

Name ______________________ Date ____________ Class ____________

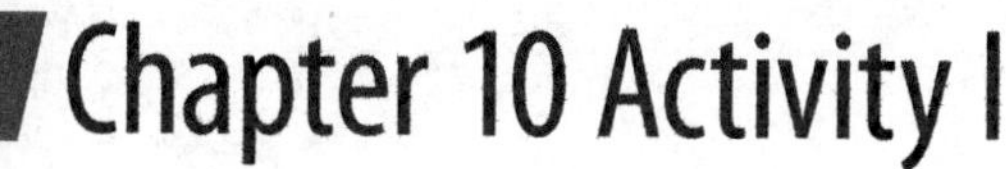

Chapter 10 Activity I

Chapter Review

Lesson 10.1 Cognitive-Behavioral Therapy

For each statement, indicate if it is True or False. If it is False, indicate how to revise the statement to make it True.

1. Talk therapies are different methods of helping people work through mental disorders.

    ____

2. Maladaptation impacts a person's ability to successfully adapt to new or difficult situations.

    ____

3. Examples of behavior therapy techniques include behavior rehearsal, biofeedback, modeling, and cognitive restructuring.

    ____

4. An example of an intermediate belief is, "I am worthy of love."

    ____

5. A defining characteristic of CBT is the interrelationship of thoughts, emotions, and behaviors.

    ____

6. By distinguishing between behaviors and thoughts, a person can deal with them more easily.

    ____

Lesson 10.2 Other Modalities

Answer the following questions.

1. _____ Compared to psychoanalytic therapy, psychodynamic therapy _____.
    A. is more focused on internal forces
    B. is more focused on external forces
    C. emphasizes social environment instead of psychosexual development
    D. emphasizes psychosexual development instead of social environment

2. _____ All of the following are characteristic of a humanistic modality *except* which?
    A. Focuses more on the journey than any end results
    B. Uses physical methods that directly influence the body
    C. Uses goals that are less specific and concrete, and less rigid
    D. Includes focus on free will, human potential, and self-discovery

3. _____ In which modality is the goal to get the client to a place where they make a conscious decision to stop certain behaviors or explore different perspectives, driven by their personal goals and free will, rather than by external pressure or shame?
    A. Biomedical
    B. Humanistic
    C. Psychodynamic
    D. Spiritual

4. _____ Which modality involves the helper and client collaborating to connect the client to a deeper meaning in the world, and often involves learning about philosophy, meditation, and recognizing there is something bigger than the self?
    A. Biomedical
    B. Humanistic
    C. Psychodynamic
    D. Spiritual

(Continued)

5. _____ Which *best* exemplifies interoceptive awareness?
   A. Exploring one's unconscious motivations
   B. Recognizing when one is feeling stressed
   C. Developing a deeper and more accurate understanding of oneself
   D. Connecting with a higher metaphysical being through prayer and contemplation

6. _____ Which is *true* of psychotropic medications?
   A. Medications universally work well for everyone with the same condition.
   B. How medications interact with an individual's brain to treat a mental disorder is fully understood by clinicians and researchers.
   C. Psychotropic medications must be approved by the Centers for Disease Control and Prevention (CDC) before they can be prescribed in the United States.
   D. It can take patients and providers time to find the right medications, the right dosage of medications, or the right balance of medications.

7. _____ A therapist who gets to know their client's situation, selects techniques they believe will be most effective, and is willing to change course and try a different technique if necessary is using which modality?
   A. Biomedical B. Humanistic C. Integrative D. Somatic

Lesson 10.3 Specialties in Mental Health

Use the terms below to match the speciality description.

Art therapy	Play therapy	Multicultural therapy
Hypnotherapy	Anger	Veterans

1. Combines the healing impact of the creative process with applied psychological theory

____

2. Helps the client reach a trance-like state of focus and heightened openness

____

3. Emphasizes the unique needs of those who have experienced war, such as adjusting to civilian life, trauma, brain injuries, and substance use disorders

____

4. Uses techniques for helping clients express negative emotions productively

____

5. Involves working with clients whose race, ethnicity, religion, income, disability status, or other social factor(s) is outside of the majority or dominant social group

____

6. Use activities such as role-play, games, or puppets to respond to clients' mental health needs

____

Answer the following questions.

7. _____ Which practice format seeks to build a community of people who are experiencing the same or similar issues or conditions?
   A. Couples B. Family C. Group D. Individual

8. _____ Which practice format allows the therapist to go deeper into issues and challenges, and gives the client more time to address their concerns and develop skills and new perspectives?
   A. Couples B. Family C. Group D. Individual

Name ______________________ Date ____________ Class ____________

CHAPTER 11

Navigating Life's Challenges

Lesson 11.1 Activity A

Understanding Trauma

Exposure to trauma can negatively affect student behavior, relationships, and academic performance. In a trauma-sensitive school, all school staff recognize and understand student responses to trauma and practices that support healing and resilience are embedded schoolwide. Read the scenarios and complete the chart and questions that follow.

Scenario 1

Maria is a 13-year-old eighth grader. She most often appears disconnected and disinterested. She fidgets, avoids eye contact, mumbles when adults ask her questions, and mostly doesn't appear to care about anything. She seems to understand the material and sometimes does well on assignments but refuses to engage with others during the school day. Teachers complain that she often puts her head down and attempts to sleep during class. This gets increasingly frustrating for adults who keep prompting Maria to sit up and engage. These power struggles frequently end with Maria either leaving the classroom or putting her head down for the remainder of the period.

Background that staff may not be aware of: Maria has an extensive history of trauma. She was removed from her home in second grade and placed with her aunt due to experiences of severe abuse and neglect. Over the years, there have been several failed attempts to reunite Maria with her mother, who struggles with addiction.

Staff Perspective (without considering trauma)	Student Perspective	Staff Perspective (with trauma glasses on)

1. What else might be important for the teachers and other school staff to know about Maria?

____

____

2. What are some potential triggers for Maria of which teachers and school staff may want to be aware?

____

____

(Continued)

3. What are some strategies teachers and school staff might consider trying with Maria?

____

____

____

Scenario 2

Jamie is a sophomore in high school and is constantly in trouble at school. He has a very short fuse and will quickly become aggressive when adults call him out on his behaviors and set limits. Jamie is particularly confrontational toward male staff. His pattern is often to begin by challenging a teacher during class—either questioning what they are doing or refusing to participate. From there, things often escalate, as Jamie becomes loud, paces around his desk, and is eventually ordered to leave the classroom. Once in the hallway, he becomes disruptive to other classrooms and has a lot of difficulty calming down.

Background that staff may not be aware of: Jamie has witnessed domestic violence and gun violence in his neighborhood, and he was bullied when he was younger. Jamie's grandmother cares for him at home but often says that she is not sure if she can continue to have him stay with her.

Staff Perspective (without considering trauma)	Student Perspective	Staff Perspective (with trauma glasses on)

4. What else might be important for the teachers and other school staff to know about Jamie?

____

____

5. What are some potential triggers for Jamie of which teachers and school staff may want to be aware?

____

____

6. What are some strategies teachers and school staff might consider trying with Jamie?

____

____

____

Name ______________________ Date ____________ Class ____________

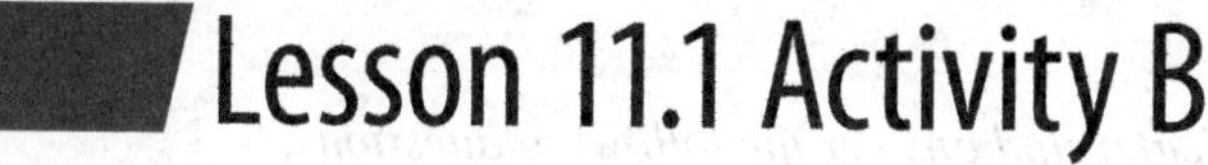

Lesson 11.1 Activity B

Bullying Statistics

Part 1

Review the facts about bullying from the Pew Research Center and answer the questions that follow.

Fact 1: About half (53%) of US teens say online harassment and online bullying are a major problem for people their age, according to a spring 2022 Center survey of teens aged 13 to 17. Another 40% say it is a minor problem, and just 6% say it is not a problem.

Fact 2: Black and Hispanic teens, those from lower-income households, and teen girls are more likely than those in other groups to view online harassment as a major problem.

Fact 3: Older teen girls are especially likely to have experienced bullying online, the survey shows. 54% of girls aged 15 to 17 have experienced at least one cyberbullying behavior asked about in the survey, compared to 44% of boys in the same age group and 41% of younger teens.

1. What age group are girls more likely to have experienced bullying online?

   ____

2. Identify at least three groups who are more likely to view online harassment as a major problem.

   ____

   ____

3. What is the difference in percentage between teens who view online harassment as a major problem and those that do not see it as a problem at all?

   ____

4. In percentage, older teen girls are how much more likely to have experienced bullying online than older teen boys?

   ____

5. As you consider your future in counseling and mental health services, who might you target with bullying and cyberbullying programming? Why?

   ____

   ____

   ____

   ____

(Continued)

Part 2

Review the graphs from surveys from the Pew Research Center and answer the following questions.

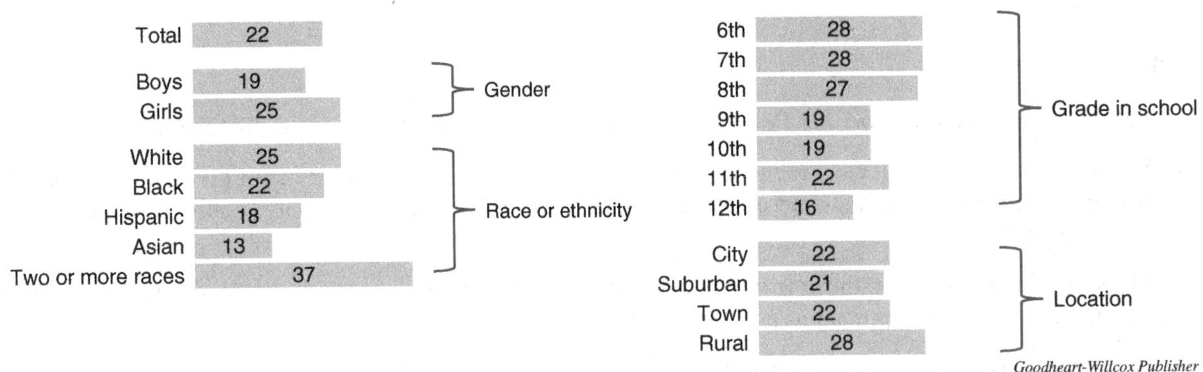

Goodheart-Willcox Publisher

1. Were boys or girls more likely to be bullied at school?

____

2. At what grade levels are students experiencing the most bullying at school?

____

3. Students from which race/ethnicity and students from which location are most impacted by bullying at school?

____

4. As you consider your future in counseling and mental health services, who might you target with school bullying programming and why? Which group had the highest instances of bullying and should be made a priority?

____

____

____

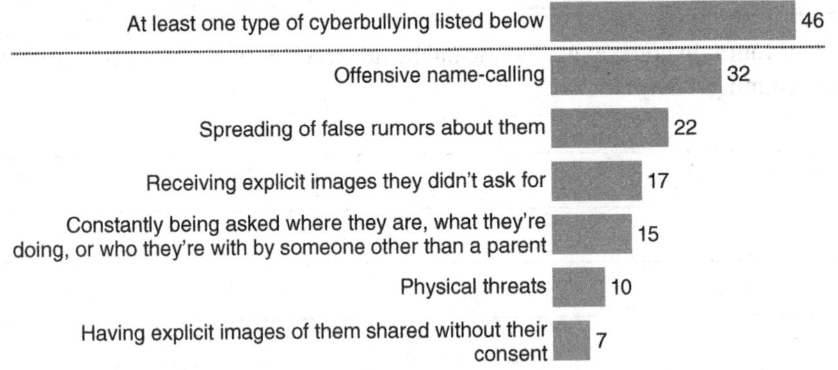

Goodheart-Willcox Publisher

5. Reviewing the graph, what are some important pieces of information you might consider if developing programming around cyberbullying?

____

____

____

____

____

Name ______________________ Date ____________ Class ____________

Lesson 11.1 Activity C

Key Terms Review

Fill in the blanks in the following statements to review the lesson's key terms.

1. Another term for positive stress, which can help increase your focus, energy, and motivation, is ______.

____

2. ______ is the reliving of a traumatic event after at least some initial adjustment to the trauma appears to have been made.

____

3. A conceptual framework for understanding how abusive relationships persist is the ______.

____

4. ______ is a cognitive disconnection between thoughts, memories, surroundings, actions, or sense of identity.

____

5. ______ is a state of worry or mental tension caused by a difficult situation.

____

6. ______ refers to harm inflicted on a partner in a romantic courting relationship.

____

7. ______ refers to those distressing events that instigate feelings of helplessness, and result in emotional dysfunction, but may not threaten life or bodily integrity.

____

8. Any disturbing experience that causes significant mental and emotional responses that have long-lasting negative effects on a person's attitudes and behavior are considered ______.

____

9. Any action by a person that causes physical harm to one or more members of their family unit is ______.

____

10. ______ is a short-term event or period in life that is stressful but will eventually pass.

____

11. A gentle, body-based, therapeutic method that heals without retraumatizing by using repetitions of a visual timeline of memories to facilitate neural integration and rapid healing is called ______.

____

12. ______ occurs when a person lives through or witnesses an event that they believe poses a threat to their life or physical integrity and safety, and experiences fear, terror, or helplessness.

____

13. ______ is a consistent sense of feeling pressured and overwhelmed over a long period of time.

____

14. Things that cause stress are known as ______.

____

15. ______ understands and considers the pervasive nature of trauma and promotes environments of healing and recovery rather than practices and services that may inadvertently retraumatize the individual.

____

Name _______________ Date _______________ Class _______________

Lesson 11.2 Activity D

Key Terms Review

Review the lesson's key terms by matching the term with the example.

1. _____ Process that involves reframing thoughts as just thoughts and not getting caught up or buying into them
2. _____ Stressful, degrading, dangerous, abusive, or damaging experiences within the context of a religious practice
3. _____ Grief marked by the need to control grief and one's environment
4. _____ Thoughts about or a preoccupation with killing oneself
5. _____ A form of psychotherapy that blends theology and behavioral sciences to help individuals or groups achieve healing and growth
6. _____ Grief with intense emotional swings and moods that people may experience after a loss
7. _____ Treatment technique that focuses on helping people begin to resolve grief by mindfully embracing it rather than fighting or masking it
8. _____ The condition of having lost a loved one to death
9. _____ The emotional distress and insecurity aroused by reminders of mortality, including one's own memories and thoughts of death
10. _____ The initial, often intense and disruptive reaction to loss
11. _____ Experience of anguish that results from a loss that is not openly acknowledged, socially mourned, or publicly supported
12. _____ A response to loss that significantly deviates from normal expectations, impedes healing, and is characterized by either delayed or absent grief or prolonged grief
13. _____ The lasting response after adjusting to loss, characterized by renewed satisfaction in ongoing life
14. _____ The experience of anguish that results from significant loss
15. _____ A critical stage or turning point at which an individual is faced with finding meaning and purpose in life and taking responsibility for their choices

A. acceptance and commitment therapy (ACT)
B. acute grief
C. bereavement
D. cognitive defusion
E. complicated grief
F. death anxiety
G. disenfranchised grief
H. existential crisis
I. grief
J. instrumental grieving
K. integrated grief
L. intuitive grieving
M. pastoral counseling
N. religious trauma
O. suicidal ideation

Name ____________________ Date ____________ Class ____________

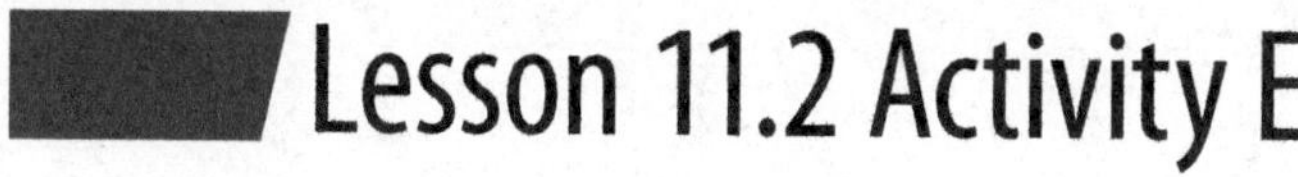

Lesson 11.2 Activity E

Types of Grief and Grieving

Complete the table below by describing each type of grief and grieving in your own words and then creating an example.

Grief/Grieving Type	Description	Example
Acute Grief		
Integrated Grief		
Complicated Grief		
Traumatic Grief		
Disenfranchised Grief		
Intuitive Grieving		
Instrumental Grieving		

Name ______________________ Date ____________ Class ____________

Lesson 11.3 Activity F

Key Terms Review

Answer the following questions to review the lesson's key terms.

1. What is the infliction of physical or emotional harm or injury to oneself?

 ____

2. What enables a person to respond effectively to new or difficult circumstances?

 ____

3. What are actions that are damaging and not in the best interest of the person performing them?

 ____

4. What is the use of cognitive and behavioral strategies to manage the demands of a situation that a person deems as beyond their capacity to handle?

 ____

5. What treatment style focuses on developing cognitive and behavioral skills to identify and prevent situations that increase the risk of relapse?

 ____

6. What inhibits a person from responding effectively to new or difficult circumstances?

 ____

7. What is the use of substances in an attempt to alleviate emotional problems?

 ____

8. What is a nonprofessional term for the sudden onset of an emotional illness that causes severe distress and significantly interferes with one's functioning?

 ____

9. A form of self-help that is not professionally guided and involves joining with others similar to oneself to explore ways to cope with life situations and problems is what?

 ____

10. What are unconscious reactions used to protect oneself from the anxiety that arises from mental conflict, external threats, and everyday problems?

 ____

11. What is it called when a person has both a substance use disorder and another mental health disorder?

 ____

12. An ability to recover from or successfully adapt to difficult or challenging life experiences is called what?

 ____

13. Addiction disorders not related to substance use are called what?

 ____

14. What type of action is seemingly innocent, accidental, or neutral, but indirectly displays an aggressive motive?

 ____

15. A cluster of physiological, behavioral, and cognitive symptoms associated with the continued use of substances despite substance-related problems and impairment is called what?

 ____

Name ______________________ Date ____________ Class ____________

Lesson 11.3 Activity G

Make the Connection

A resource developed and operated by the US Department of Veterans Affairs (VA), Make the Connection aims to reduce barriers and stigma associated with mental health challenges that may prevent veterans from seeking mental health care.

Part 1

Review the reflection questions below and then go to the Make the Connection website. Use the advanced filtering tool to view videos about substance use, alcohol use, and gambling. View as many videos as you like to respond to the reflection questions.

1. What emotions came up for you while listening to the veterans' stories?

____

____

____

2. What did you learn about substance use disorders and the people affected by them?

____

____

____

3. What did you learn about the experience of veterans?

____

____

____

4. How can the videos you watched help people dealing with substance use disorders?

____

____

____

5. What is something you heard that surprised or intrigued you?

____

____

____

6. Did your perceptions of substance use or gambling change? If so, how?

____

____

____

(Continued)

Part 2

View other veterans' stories on Make the Connection that relate to what interests you. There are stories about adjustment disorder, mood disorders, social withdrawal, schizophrenia, PTSD, suicide, eating problems, and flashbacks, among others. Record any takeaways or points of interest you gleaned from the stories.

Name ______________________ Date __________ Class __________

Chapter 11 Activity H

Chapter Review

Lesson 11.1 Stress and Trauma

Indicate which stress management technique each person is applying. You can review these techniques in Figure 11.2 and Figure 11.3.

1. To relieve muscle tension caused by stress, Jerome closes his eyes and breathes deeply. Starting from his feet and moving up to his head, Jerome gently tightens and then relaxes muscle groups.

   ____

2. Feeling stressed by some upsetting news, Isabell uses human touch to release oxytocin, lower blood pressure, and relax.

   ____

3. Nene closes her eyes and imagines being in the back seat of her grandmother's car. She imagines smelling the leather upholstery, the cushy, smooth ride, and the sound of her grandmother humming church hymns, and she quickly begins to feel less stress.

   ____

4. No matter how busy Jamie gets at work, they make time to go play soccer with their friends Thursday evenings.

   ____

5. When Carrie's friend calls her, upset because of something her partner said to her, Carrie stops what she is doing and makes sure she is fully present to listen to her.

   ____

Answer the following questions.

6. _____ All of the following are symptoms of posttraumatic stress disorder, *except* which?
   A. Engaging in activities or revisiting places that recall the traumatic event
   B. Reexperiencing the trauma in painful recollections, flashbacks, or recurring dreams or nightmares
   C. Diminished responsiveness, including emotional numbness, disinterest in significant activities, and detachment and isolation from others
   D. An exaggerated startle response, disturbed sleep, and difficulty concentrating or remembering

7. _____ What mental phenomenon helps during the traumatic event, but can also prevent the person from recovering from the trauma by preventing them from processing the experience and returning to psychological safety?
   A. Dissociation B. Eustress C. Flashbacks D. Survivor's guilt

8. _____ Muhamed is the only boy in his family. Through therapy, he comes to understand that his emotional and social needs were often not treated as important as his sisters' needs. This likely contributed to his avoidant behaviors. What does this experience exemplify?
   A. Eustress B. Acute stress C. Big "T" trauma D. Little "t" trauma

9. _____ Which of the following *best* exemplifies trauma-informed care?
   A. Focusing on practices and services that retraumatize the individual
   B. Training all staff to view people's behaviors through a trauma lens
   C. Focusing on the outcomes of trauma, rather than the environment
   D. Training clinicians to understand PTSD

(Continued)

10. _____ Which *best* characterizes the mental health effects of bullying?
   A. Students who are bullied are more likely to attend school.
   B. The antisocial behaviors of students who bully others are less likely to escalate.
   C. Students who witness bullying feel stress from the fear of retaliation or inaction.
   D. Bullying decreases the likelihood a person will experience depression, anxiety, and low self-esteem.

Lesson 11.2 Death and Grief

For each statement, indicate if the statement is True or False. If False, indicate how to correct the statement to make it True.

1. The somatic modality can helpful insights and approaches to helping people address their concerns or issues around death.

   ____

2. An existential crisis can describe any psychological or moral crisis that causes a person to question human existence, including challenging their own previously held beliefs or worldviews.

   ____

3. If a counselor wants to incorporate spirituality and religion into their work, they must first thoroughly explore their own religious and spiritual beliefs, or lack thereof.

   ____

4. Counselors must be trained pastoral counselors and be experts on their client's faith to incorporate religion and spirituality into the therapy they provide.

   ____

5. Research suggests exposure to suicide-related information, resources, and discussion leads to increases in suicidal ideation and a higher likelihood of engaging in suicidal behavior.

   ____

6. Talking about wanting to die, having great guilt or shame, or being a burden to others, including expressing unbearable emotion or physical pain, is a warning sign of suicide.

   ____

7. If someone admits to you that they are thinking about suicide, one important step is to not leave them alone and to stay with them until you can get them to a caregiver, caring adult, or trained professional.

   ____

8. Bereavement is the experience of anguish that results from a significant loss.

   ____

9. There is a typical response to loss, and people grieve by moving through the stages in order.

   ____

10. One goal of acceptance and commitment therapy (ACT) is to develop a self-as-context mindset that frames experiences, thoughts, and feelings as ever-changing content that is part of their life journey, but not who they are.

   ____

(Continued)

Name ________________________________

Lesson 11.3 Coping and Substance Use Disorders

Match the coping strategy with the orientation.

Avoidant	**Problem-Focused**
Approach	**Emotion-Focused**

1. Using drugs or alcohol to escape

____

2. Talking with others about stressors

____

3. Asking for advice from others on what to do

____

4. Finding the positive

____

Match the defense mechanism with the example

Anticipation	**Identification**	**Sublimation**
Humor	**Regression**	**Fantasy**
Reaction Formation	**Displacement**	**Rationalization**
Denial	**Projection**	

5. A man who feels insecure about his masculinity mocks another man for displaying perceived feminine behavior.

____

6. Worried about an upcoming first date, a person imagines romantic experience worthy of a major motion picture.

____

7. A person with a substance use disorder praises the virtue of temperance.

____

8. Someone writes poetry and creates music to process negative emotions and thoughts.

____

9. A person feeling like a failure for struggling to pay their bills starts taking their frustration out on people in their family and blaming them for being unable to find a job that pays well.

____

10. A person who fears their demanding, merciless, and driven boss adopts similar personality traits in hopes of avoiding negative consequences.

____

11. In preparation for a difficult conversation with one's boss at work, someone thinks through likely and worst-case scenarios and how they can react professionally but assertively.

____

(Continued)

Answer the following questions.

12. List three factors that contribute to a person's resiliency.

____

____

____

13. _____ All of the following are symptoms of a substance use disorder *except* which?
    A. Loss of control
    B. Risky use
    C. Shame
    D. Social impairment

14. _____ The modern perspective on substance use disorders reframes them as _____.
    A. a medical condition rather than a mental disorder
    B. a mental disorder rather than a medical condition
    C. more of a personal failing of the individual and less as a mental disorder and medical condition
    D. both a mental disorder and medical condition and less of a personal failing of the individual

15. _____ Co-occurring disorders occur when a person has _____.
    A. any two mental disorders
    B. any two medical conditions
    C. a mental disorder and a substance use disorder
    D. any combination of a mental disorder and medical condition

16. _____ Which of the following is a risk factor for developing a substance use disorder?
    A. Fewer adverse childhood experiences
    B. Earlier age of initiation of use
    C. Ethnic and racial identity
    D. Socioeconomic class

17. _____ A facility where the person lives for a period of time, and which may or may not allow them to learn or work in the community, describes which practice setting of substance use disorder treatment?
    A. Inpatient
    B. Outpatient
    C. Relapse prevention
    D. Residential

Name ______________________ Date ____________ Class ____________

CHAPTER 12 Living with Integrity

Lesson 12.1 Activity A

Key Terms Review

Fill in the blanks in the following statements to review the lesson's key terms.

1. ______ describes the mental discomfort that results from one element in a person's cognitive system contradicting another.

   ____

2. ______ is a person's subjective perception of their capability to perform in a given situation.

   ____

3. A(n) ______ is continuously learning, is willing to try new things, and believes that people's abilities can change and develop.

   ____

4. The ______ is a process model grounded in the theory that changing health behaviors takes time, effective interventions vary based on the stages, and there are multiple outcomes at each stage.

   ____

5. ______ is the degree to which a person is receptive to an experience or activity, such as mental health treatment.

   ____

6. ______ means that someone can do something without depending on others.

   ____

7. A(n) ______ believes abilities are innate and unchangeable.

   ____

8. ______ is the power to take action without being confined by fear so that one may live a meaningful life.

   ____

9. ______ occurs when a person increases the consistency between elements of their cognitive system.

   ____

10. The impulse or desire to investigate, observe, or gather information, particularly when the subject is new or interesting, is called ______.

    ____

11. A sense of safety and confidence without experiencing fear, worry, and anxiety is called ______.

    ____

12. A theory which suggests that just affirming something you value about yourself can reduce dissonance is called ______.

    ____

13. ______ refers to a state of mind that influences how a person thinks about and approaches their goal-directed activities in ways that either promote or interfere with optimal functioning.

    ____

Name ______________________________ Date ______________ Class ____________

Lesson 12.1 Activity B

Stages of Change Story

For this activity, write a story where the main character works through three of the six stages of change sequentially (stages 1-3, 2-4, 3-5, or 4-6). It should be clear which three stages the main character is moving through. The topic of the change can be anything related to mental, social, or emotional health.

Name ______________________ Date ____________ Class ____________

Lesson 12.2 Activity C

Key Terms Review

Part 1

Review the lesson's key terms by matching the term with the example.

1. _____ A feeling people experience when they have fallen short of their values
2. _____ An act of emotional exposure that can foster positive mental health outcomes
3. _____ A process of feeling increasingly ashamed of oneself to the point that one is unable to control or stop their self-loathing
4. _____ A distancing act of pity for another person's situation
5. _____ A thought or state of mind that a person holds as the absolute truth and that stops them from doing certain things
6. _____ The painful emotional reaction to feeling one is unworthy of love and belonging
7. _____ Knowing that, even with your flaws, you are enough
8. _____ The act of connecting with someone in pain and communicating through action that they are not alone

A. empathy
B. guilt
C. limiting belief
D. shame
E. shame spiral
F. sympathy
G. vulnerability
H. worthiness

Part 2

Match the example of a limiting belief to one of the following categories.

1. _____ I am too old to apply for that job.
2. _____ The city is too dangerous to go to.
3. _____ Jill is too young to be a responsible babysitter.
4. _____ Doctors can't be trusted.
5. _____ I am too shy to run for the school board.
6. _____ People in this town are the problem.
7. _____ Reggie is too weak to do this kind of work.

A. about oneself
B. about others
C. about the world

Name ______________________ Date ______________ Class __________

Lesson 12.2 Activity D

Personal Reflection

Respond to the following prompts and questions to reflect on the art of living.

1. Complete this sentence: Vulnerability is…

2. List some ways that people may protect themselves from rejection, heartbreak, embarrassment, and criticism.

3. How does connection enable a person to be more vulnerable?

4. Write down a limiting belief that someone you know possesses. (Do not identify the person.) Write down some questions that would challenge that limiting belief.

5. How do shame or the fear of shame limit a person's vulnerability and authenticity?

6. Have you ever experienced shame? What did it feel like?

7. Think of empathy as a skill that can be developed. What are some ways that you could improve your ability to practice empathy?

8. Why do you think telling your shame story combats shame?

9. Inevitably, people who practice the art of living will make mistakes. Practicing self-compassion helps improve one's resiliency to these mistakes. Research exercises and practices to build self-compassion. Jot down some that you may be willing to try below.

Name ______________________ Date ____________ Class ____________

Lesson 12.2 Activity E

Recognizing Empathy

Most attempts at empathy are very well-intentioned, but they end up passing over the person's emotional distress, which is what they are dealing with in the moment they are vulnerable enough to share their struggle. There may or may not be time later if you want to offer advice or share a similar experience you have encountered. Initially, however, you need to empathize. This means imagining yourself in their situation, offering connection, actively listening, and validating their emotions.

The following terms describe failures to communicate empathy (and one that describes true empathy). For each term, write a scenario as an example of an interaction between two people showing this failure of empathy. Finally, write a scenario between two people that demonstrates successful communication of empathy.

Empathy Fail	Description	Scenario
Advising	*Offering advice that the person can apply to their situation*	
One-Upping	*Sharing an experience that you perceive as worse than theirs*	
Consoling	*Comforting a person by trying to make them feel better*	
Explaining	*Offering excuses or explanations*	
Shutting Down	*Abruptly ending the conversation by redirecting or minimizing*	
Correcting	*Deflecting by pointing out the person's mistakes*	
Fixing It	*Swooping in to solve the problem for the person*	
Storytelling	*Sharing an experience that relates to the person's situation*	
Educating	*Trying to teach a concept, behavior, or information that you perceive as being helpful*	
Interrogating	*Asking several questions to analyze the person's situation*	
Sympathizing	*Expressing pity for someone and their situation*	
Empathizing	*Connecting with someone in pain and communicating through action that they are not alone*	

Name ______________________ Date ______________ Class ____________

Lesson 12.3 Activity F

Key Terms Review

Answer the following questions to review the lesson's key terms.

1. What occurs when joy triggers worry or dread that is motivated by a desire to protect oneself from the vulnerability of allowing oneself to feel joy?

   ____

2. A state of optimal experience arising from intense involvement in an activity that is enjoyable is what?

   ____

3. What provides an approach to wellness that emphasizes self-compassion, lifelong learning, and taking action to achieve a more joyful, fulfilled life?

   ____

4. A sense of thankfulness and happiness in response to receiving something is called what?

   ____

5. What is the pressure to express only positive emotions and suppress negative emotions, reactions, or experiences?

   ____

6. What describes the practice of taking steps to improve one's well-being?

   ____

7. A pleasurable feeling based on circumstances is called what?

   ____

8. What is the amount of sleep that you need to make up for lost sleep called?

   ____

9. What is a mood or attitude that promotes resilience, peace, and connection regardless of circumstances?

   ____

10. What is the cognitive ability to sustain awareness of one's internal states and surroundings in the present moment?

    ____

11. What includes both an emergency, short-term psychological intervention for people experiencing a mental health crisis, and a brief use of psychotherapy or counseling to alleviate the immediate distress of a highly disruptive experience?

    ____

12. What is a field of theory and research that focuses on the positive emotions, states and strengths, and institutions that make life most worth living?

    ____

Name ______________________ Date ____________ Class ____________

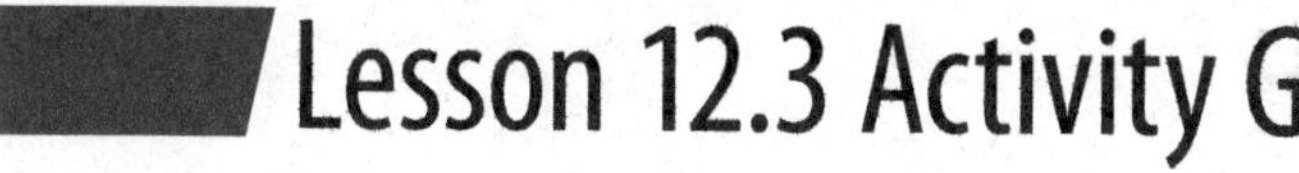

Lesson 12.3 Activity G

Wellness Self-Assessment

Part 1

Refer to Figure 12.15. For each of the SPIRE dimensions of wellness, self-assess your health in that dimension on a scale of one to 6, with 6 being very healthy and 1 being the greatest opportunity for improvement.

Dimension of Well-Being	Self-Assessment Score (1–6)
Spiritual	
Physical	
Intellectual	
Rational	
Emotional	

Part 2

Referring to your self-assessment, identify two dimensions you would like to work on improving over the next 6 months. Complete a table for each dimension.

Prompt	Response
Dimension #1	
Describe how you think you would feel in 6 months after improving in this dimension.	
What are some specific activities you can do to improve your wellness in this dimension? ***(Hint: you can use the reflective questions in Figure 12.15)***	
What are some specific resources that could help you improve your wellness in this dimension? ***(Hint: people you could talk with, specific podcasts or books)***	

Prompt	Response
Dimension #2	
Describe how you think you would feel in 6 months after improving in this dimension.	
What are some specific activities you can do to improve your wellness in this dimension? ***(Hint: you can use the reflective questions in Figure 12.15)***	
What are some specific resources that could help you improve your wellness in this dimension? ***(Hint: people you could talk with, specific podcasts or books)***	

Name ______________________ Date ______________ Class ______________

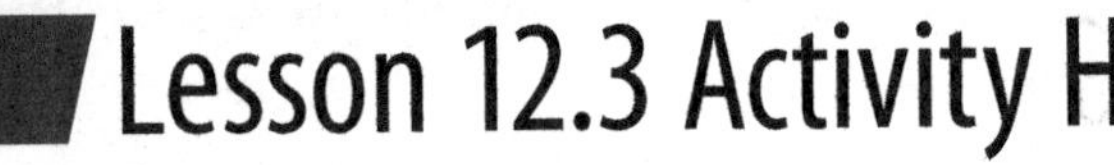

Lesson 12.3 Activity H

Practicing Gratitude

Part 1

Write five things you appreciated this week. Use complete sentences.

1. ____

2. ____

3. ____

4. ____

5. ____

Part 2

Think about a challenge you have overcome. Write that challenge and how you grew and overcame the challenge. Use complete sentences.

____

Part 3

Write an example of a thank-you note to one of your teachers or school personnel. After writing the example, review with a classmate and consider utilizing the message to write a thank-you card to the teacher or school personnel.

____

Name ______________________ Date ____________ Class ____________

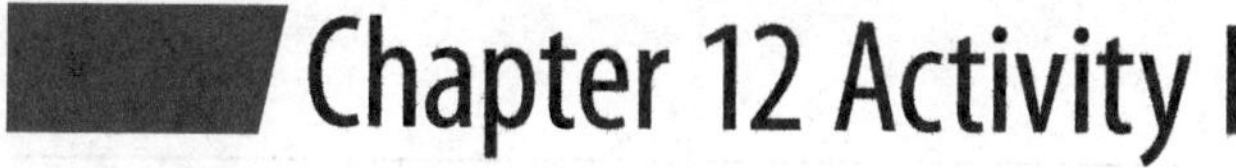

Chapter 12 Activity I

Chapter Review

Lesson 12.1 Readiness for Change

For each description below, identify the stage of change and rank the stages in order:

Rank	Stage	Description
		A person is motivated to change and actively involved in taking steps to change by using various techniques
		A person considers changing
		The changes become less novel and more integrated into a person's "new normal"
		People have committed to making a change and engage in actions to learn more and understand the changes necessary
		A person has no intention of changing; they may be unaware or under-aware of their problems

Use the mindsets listed below to answer the following questions.

Deliberative	**Fixed**	**Growth**
Implemental	**Prevention**	**Promotion**

1. Which two mindsets describe how a person considers information when making decisions?

____

2. Which mindset engages in continuously learning, is willing to try new things, and develop new skills?

____

3. Which two mindsets describe a person's core drive or motivation in their work?

____

4. Which mindset believes abilities are innate and unchangeable?

____

Lesson 12.2 The Art of Living

For each statement, indicate if it is True or False. If False, explain how to correct the statement to make it True.

1. Connection is an essential need of all people; disconnection leads to freedom.

____

2. Everyone is worthy of love, belonging, and joy.

____

3. Authentically engaging in the world requires defensiveness and impenetrable emotional walls.

____

(Continued)

4. Vulnerability is a weakness.

____

5. Connection serves as the best resource for countering the fear, rejection, and criticism of practicing vulnerability.

____

6. True, deep connection with others does not require a person to practice vulnerability.

____

7. Practicing worthiness can be challenging for someone with an abundance mindset.

____

8. Limiting beliefs often focus on oneself, others (also known as prejudice), or how the world works.

____

9. Limiting beliefs prevent judgment of others and oneself, making it more difficult for a person to experience true authenticity and deep connection.

____

10. Shame resilience theory (SRT) provides a method for managing and overcoming shame.

____

Lesson 12.3 Positive Psychology and Wellness

Answer the following questions.

1. _____ All of the following characterize the psychological concept of flow, *except* ______.
   A. peak extrinsic motivation
   B. loss of self-consciousness and temporal awareness
   C. alignment of a person's skills to the demands of the task
   D. total control, effortlessness, and complete concentration on the immediate situation

2. _____ Happiness is a pleasurable feeling based on circumstances, while joy ______.
   A. occurs regardless of one's current situation
   B. depends on external factors
   C. is cultivated relatively quickly
   D. results from fun activities

3. _____ "How do you practice and cultivate creativity?" is an appropriate reflection question for which SPIRE dimension of well-being?
   A. Spiritual B. Physical C. Intellectual D. Relational

4. _____ "What are your shame triggers?" is an appropriate reflection question for which SPIRE dimension of well-being?
   A. Physical B. Intellectual C. Relational D. Emotional

5. _____ Exercises that quiet the brain and center it in the present moment are which type of wellness practice?
   A. Gratitude B. Journaling C. Mindfulness D. Sleep and rest

6. _____ Which wellness practice is grounded in positive psychology and shown to help people feel more positive emotions, enjoy good experiences, improve health, deal with adversity, and build strong relationships?
   A. Gratitude B. Journaling C. Mindfulness D. Sleep and rest

7. _____ Which wellness practice supports positive mood, ability to learn and remember, and executive functioning skills?
   A. Gratitude B. Journaling C. Mindfulness D. Sleep and rest

Name ______________________ Date ____________ Class ____________

CHAPTER 13

School and Career Counseling

Lesson 13.1 Activity A

Key Terms Review

Fill in the blanks in the following statements to review the lesson's key terms.

1. ______ is when students have the knowledge, skills, resources, and attitudes to effectively assume adult roles and responsibilities.

   ____

2. The resources a program uses in its activities and services are called ______.

   ____

3. The ______ include the learning strategies, self-management skills, and social skills commonly associated with being a successful student.

   ____

4. The ______ relate to students' psychosocial attitudes or beliefs about themselves in relation to academic work.

   ____

5. The ______ was established to provide a national, unifying professional organization for school counselors.

   ____

6. ______ is when students have the knowledge, skills, resources, and attitudes to access the postsecondary education and training option that aligns with their career goals.

   ____

7. ______ are procedures and approaches students use to help them in the cognitive work of thinking, remembering, or learning.

   ____

8. ______ is when students have the knowledge, skills, resources, and attitudes to make their career goals and plans a reality.

   ____

9. ______ are students' abilities to regulate their own behaviors, thoughts, and emotions in a productive way.

   ____

10. The outcomes and impact of a program's activities and services are called ______.

    ____

11. ______ are acceptable behaviors students use to improve the social interactions with peers and adults.

    ____

Name ______________________ Date ____________ Class ________

Lesson 13.1 Activity B

History of School Counseling Timeline

For each letter on the timeline, explain the milestone or evolution that took place in the formation of the school counseling profession.

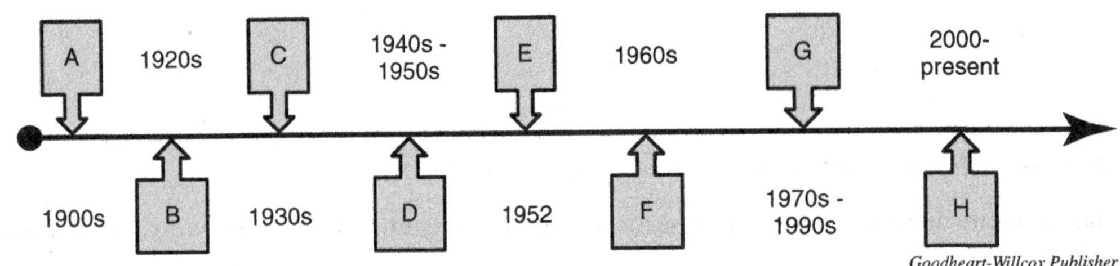

Goodheart-Willcox Publisher

A. ____

B. ____

C. ____

D. ____

E. ____

F. ____

G. ____

H. ____

Name ______________________ Date ______________ Class ______________

Lesson 13.2 Activity C

Key Terms Review

Review the lesson's key terms by matching the term with the example.

1. _____ Blend of individual and group therapy techniques with teaching methods
2. _____ A school and career counseling practice that involves conferring directly with teachers, caregivers, administrators, and other helping professionals
3. _____ A willingness to change or compromise
4. _____ The maturation of a person's ability to manage emotions and learn and apply interpersonal skills
5. _____ The number of students for each school counselor in the school building
6. _____ The maturation of a person's ability to learn
7. _____ A counseling intervention used to empower non-counselors with knowledge, skills, and resources to address counseling and mental health issues in non-counseling settings
8. _____ The process of organizing, planning, and controlling time spent on different activities
9. _____ Short-term, goal-focused counseling technique that aims to help clients change by creating solutions rather than focusing on problems

A. academic development
B. consultation
C. flexibility
D. psychoeducation
E. social/emotional development
F. solution-focused brief therapy (SFBT)
G. student-to-school-counselor ratio
H. time management
I. training

Name ______________________________ Date ______________ Class ______________

Lesson 13.2 Activity D

Student-to-School-Counselor Ratio

The ASCA recommends a ratio of 250 students for every 1 school counselor. Research your school and state ratios and answer the following questions.

1. What is your school or school system's student-to-school-counselor ratio?

____

2. What is your state average for student-to-school-counselor ratio?

____

3. Compare and contrast your school and state ratios to the recommended ratio from the ASCA.

____

____

4. What are some challenges of having a high student-to-school-counselor ratio?

____

____

____

5. What are some benefits of having a lower student-to-school-counselor ratio?

____

____

____

6. What are some reasons a school may want to consider a smaller than recommended student-to-school-counselor ratio?

____

____

____

____

____

Name ______________________ Date ______________ Class ______________

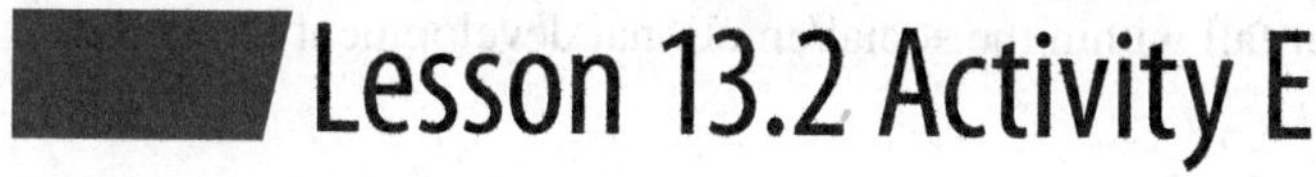

Lesson 13.2 Activity E

School Counselor Informational Interview

Part 1

Interview a school counselor to learn more about the skills and techniques they use in their job. Use the template below to track your notes about their responses.

1. What grade level(s) do you work with? What makes being a school counselor for this age group unique, compared to other age groups?

____

____

____

2. What do you enjoy most about your job as a school counselor?

____

____

____

____

____

3. What challenges do you experience in your job? How do you try to overcome or minimize them?

____

____

____

4. What school counseling theories or techniques do you use most?

____

____

____

____

____

5. I learned that school counselors plan, implement, and evaluate a comprehensive school counseling program. Could you tell me a little about that process from your perspective?

____

____

____

____

____

____

(Continued)

6. What types of activities or services do you provide that fall within the social/emotional development domain of school counseling?

____

____

____

7. . . . the academic development domain?

____

____

____

8. . . . the career development domain?

____

____

____

9. Student-generated question:

____

____

____

Part 2

Meet with a classmate and go over the responses each of you received. If possible, meet with a student who interviewed a school counselor who works with a different age group (elementary, middle, or high school). Note the things that were similar and different from each of your interviews in the table below.

Similarities	Differences

Extension Activity

Using thank-you notes or supplies provided by your teacher, write a thank-you note to the school counselor you interviewed.

Name ______________________ Date ____________ Class ____________

Lesson 13.3 Activity F

Key Terms Review

Answer the following questions to review the lesson's key terms.

1. What is the sequence of career-related choices and transitions made over the life span?

____

2. What is defined as having successfully completed the developmental goals and tasks during the stage at which one would optimally be able to do so?

____

3. A service that involves counseling or research on behalf of a client for the purpose of directing them to other agencies or organizations that provide assistance and services is called what?

____

4. An application or software program that allows people to explore careers, labor market information, and training and education requirements is called what?

____

5. A person interviews someone working in an occupation or field of interest to glean information that can be used in career planning in what?

____

6. What is the process of helping an individual or a group of clients make informed career choices and transitions?

____

7. What is the process of ongoing data collection and making changes to products, services, or processes with an emphasis on incremental and ongoing improvement?

____

8. What formal career assessment category helps clients identify and understand their interest patterns or themes?

____

9. What is a theory which suggests that individuals and occupations have unique characteristics that can be measured and then matched to create a good fit that satisfies both the individual and the employer?

____

10. What is a process used to enable people with mental and physical disabilities to overcome barriers to accessing, maintaining, or returning to employment?

____

11. What are informal assessment activities in which clients choose between two or more alternatives in response to a specific question?

____

12. The data about the supply and demand for employment is called what?

____

Name ______________________ Date ____________ Class ____________

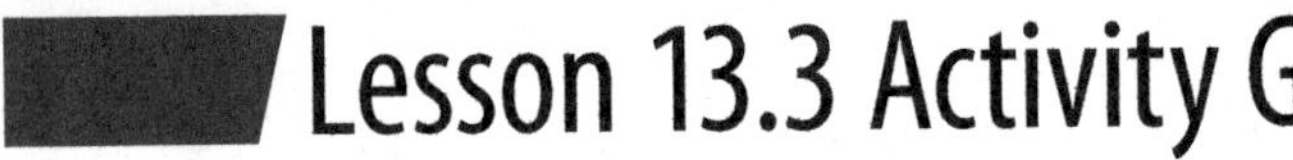

Lesson 13.3 Activity G

Career Development Theories

Research the career development theories below to complete the following activities and answer the following questions.

Theory	Theorist	Elements/Models
Trait-and-Factor Theory	John Holland	Holland Codes, consistency, congruence
Social Learning Theory	John Krumboltz	Role models, positive reinforcement, emphasis on teaching people to navigate career decisions, happenstance events
Career Development Theory	Donald Super	Self-concept, work values, life span stage, career maturity, life space, life-career rainbow, archway of career determinants
Transition Theory	Nancy Schlossberg	Focus on points in time when change is occurring, coping and adaptation, 4-S Model

Trait-and-Factor Theory

1. Go to O*Net Online, navigate to the Interest Profiler, and take the assessment. Record your scores for each Holland Code category.
   A. _____ Realistic
   B. _____ Investigative
   C. _____ Artistic
   D. _____ Social
   E. _____ Enterprising
   F. _____ Conventional
2. On O*Net Online, search for the following occupations and indicate their Holland Codes.
   A. _____ Educational, Guidance, and Career Counselors and Advisors
   B. _____ Mental Health Counselors
   C. _____ Clinical Neuropsychologists
   D. _____ Social and Human Service Assistants
   E. _____ Art Therapists
   F. _____ Electricians
   G. _____ Human Resource Managers
   H. _____ Veterinarians
3. How do your results compare to those of the occupations listed above? Which, if any, align closely with your results? Which of them differ?

____

____

____

____

4. What are your thoughts on your results? What do you agree or disagree with?

____

____

(Continued)

Name ______________________________

Social Learning Theory

1. Imagine working with a client in college who has a lot of anxiety about job interviews. Applying Krumboltz's social learning theory, how could you help them?

2. Why would Krumboltz see value in helping clients find positive role models?

3. Krumboltz introduced the concept of "unplanned happenstance," which suggests that a person should develop the ability to find opportunities in unplanned events. Think about a time in your life when a happenstance event provided an opportunity. List some ideas on how you might help a client respond to happenstance events.

Super's Career Development Theory

1. Imagine working with a client who could not work in an occupation that aligns with their interests. What would Super suggest as a way to use those interests?

Search online for Super's "Archway of Career Determinants." This graphic was Super's last contribution to the field and was intended to summarize his life's work. Note that biography and geography form the base of all career decisions. Use this graphic to answer the following questions.

2. What components of biography contribute to a person's career decisions?

3. What components of geography contribute to a person's career decisions?

4. What is at the keystone (center) of the arch? What element supports the keystone on either side?

(Continued)

5. Why do you think Super designed the archway of career determinants this way? What was he trying to convey? Does it, or parts of it, remind you of any other theories you have learned about?

____

____

____

____

Transition Theory

Situation
• How much change is required in roles, relationships, and routines? • Is this transition expected or unexpected? • How much control does the person have over the transition? What are their options? • How long will this transition last? • What else is going on?
Self
• Where is the person's locus of control? • What skills and adaptive behaviors (such as stress management, decision-making, or assertiveness) does the person possess? • How has the person navigated transitions in the past? • What is their resilience like?
Supports
• Are there friends and family who can help through the transition? • Is there enough money or other material resources to get through the transition? • What agencies or other service providers exist to provide support through the transition?
Strategies
• How can the situation be viewed more positively? • What inner resources could be further developed through this transition? • Are there support people or agencies to whom you can refer the client? • What are some options to move the client out of this situation? Which option seems to be the best? • What action steps should be implemented to initiate the selected option?

1. How could working through a career transition cycle with a counselor using Schlossberg's theory help the client in the future or in other domains of life?

____

____

____

____

2. Describe the type of client you think would most benefit from a counselor using Schlossberg's theory. What is their self-confidence (or self-efficacy) like? What barriers might they face?

____

____

____

____

Name ______________________________ Date ______________ Class ____________

Chapter 13 Activity H

Chapter Review

Lesson 13.1 Professional School Counseling

For each statement, indicate if it is True or False. If False, explain how to correct the statement to make it True.

1. The first major shift in the formation of school counseling was from only focusing on personal adjustment counseling to including more vocational guidance.

   ____

2. During the 1930s, the concept of guidance services emerged and is considered part of a broader student services department of nonteaching and nonadministrative school roles.

   ____

3. During the 1940s and 1950s, school counseling took root in elementary schools.

   ____

4. Modern school counseling programs use the American Psychological Association's National Model, providing consistency to standardize school counseling programs across the United States.

   ____

5. Compared to the concept of "school counselors," guidance counselors are proactive to student needs and informed by data.

   ____

6. Many professional helpers and human services leaders use program logic models to help with program planning, implementation, management, evaluation, and reporting.

   ____

7. Program logic models map out program inputs, activities, and outputs, and encourage using data and evaluating outputs only.

   ____

8. Academic development, one of the three domains of school counseling, includes activities that help students manage emotions and learn and apply interpersonal skills.

   ____

Lesson 13.2 School Counseling Skills and Techniques

For each statement, answer either "Yes" or "No" to indicate whether it would be appropriate for a school counselor to perform that task.

1. _____ Provide coverage or substitute in classrooms for absent teachers.
2. _____ Discipline students or assign disciplinary consequences.
3. _____ Consult with career and technical education (CTE) teachers to support students' career development.
4. _____ Manage student data and records like transcripts and discipline records.
5. _____ Plan and implement a psychoeducation skills training on test-taking strategies for a small group of students with test anxiety.

(Continued)

6. _____ Provide long-term counseling for psychological disorders.

7. _____ Consult with the school social worker, caregiver, and administrator to intervene when a student is in crisis.

8. _____ Manage the individualized education plans (IEPs) of exceptional learners.

Lesson 13.3 Career Development and Counseling

Answer the following questions.

1. _____ Founded in 1913, what professional association provides professional development, publications, standards, and advocacy to practitioners and educators who inspire and empower individuals to achieve their career and life goals?
   A. APA B. ASCA C. NASW D. NCDA

2. _____ A defined set of work tasks commonly performed for the purpose of making a particular product or performing a specific service *best* describes which term?
   A. Career B. Industry C. Job D. Occupation

3. _____ Robbie is helping a client evaluate different career paths by helping them understand how demand may change based on historical trends. Robbie is using which type of labor market information?
   A. Number of job openings for an occupation
   B. Average salaries or wages for an occupation
   C. Projected growth of an industry or occupation
   D. Number of firms or establishments in an industry

4. _____ Compared to a program's service population, the target population are the _____.
   A. special populations who are disadvantaged in some way
   B. people who receive benefits from the program
   C. special populations who access the program
   D. people for whom the program is designed

5. _____ Charlotte is a single parent and is taking into consideration which occupations and career paths would offer growth opportunities and would allow her to support her two children financially and care for her children when they are not in school. This *best* exemplifies which client factor?
   A. Strengths B. Preferences C. Interests D. Needs

6. _____ Which component of the SMART goal model is missing in the following goal? "I will research the three careers we discussed today and identify one about which I would like to learn more."
   A. Measurable B. Achievable C. Realistic D. Timely

7. _____ Josh wants to help his client explore the things she cares deeply about so that she may find a career that fulfills her and gives her life meaning. Which type of career assessment should he use?
   A. Abilities test
   B. Interest inventory
   C. Skill inventory
   D. Work value inventory

8. _____ According to John L. Holland's theory, which client would *most likely* experience more instability in their career due to their varied interests?
   A. Client A: Realistic-Investigative
   B. Client B: Artistic-Conventional
   C. Client C: Social-Enterprising
   D. Client D: Enterprising-Realistic

9. _____ A mental health counselor is working with a client who is in his mid-60s and struggling with pressure from his partner to retire. The client is having difficulty disengaging in his worker life role and engaging in a different lifestyle that includes more leisure, family, and community activities. This *best* exemplifies whose career development theory?
   A. Donald Super
   B. John Holland
   C. John Krumboltz
   D. Nancy Schlossberg

Name ______________________ Date ______________ Class ____________

CHAPTER 14

The Helping Relationship

Lesson 14.1 Activity A

Key Terms Review

Fill in the blanks in the following statements to review the lesson's key terms.

1. A(n) _____ is an approach to psychoanalysis that sees the client as a whole person in need of validation, empathy, and warmth and the counselor as a whole person with values, beliefs, experiences, and feelings.

____

2. _____ is when one person assists another in exploring feelings, gaining insight, and making changes in their life.

____

3. _____ is the expression of enthusiasm, affection, or kindness.

____

4. _____ is the quality of being real, honest, and sincere.

____

5. A close and harmonious relationship in which the people or groups involved understand each other's feelings and ideas and communicate well is _____.

____

6. A behavior that is immediate and without conscious thought, often driven by emotions, is _____.

____

7. _____ is the firm belief in the reliability, truth, ability, or strength of someone.

____

8. _____ occurs when clients rely too much on helpers for support and feel unable to explore feelings or make changes in their lives without assistance from the helper.

____

9. _____ is the ability to withhold criticism; believe a person's opinions, experiences, and feelings; and meet them where they are.

____

10. _____ implies thoughtful action that considers immediate and long-term outcomes in the context of the situation.

____

11. _____ is a conscious effort to acknowledge and honor difficult situations and emotions.

____

12. _____ means that a person's actions are aligned with their values and desires, despite external pressures.

____

13. When counselors are _____, they offer someone confidence and hope.

____

Name ______________________ Date ______________ Class ____________

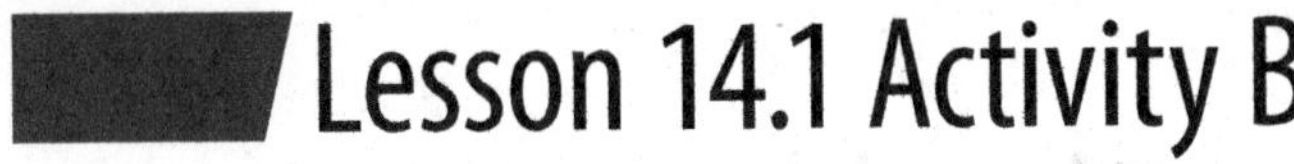

Lesson 14.1 Activity B

Person-to-Person Relationship

Carol Rogers promoted three essential qualities of effective counselors: congruence/genuineness, unconditional positive regard, and empathetic understanding. These qualities are embedded in Figures 14.2 and 14.3.

Part 1

For each column, write three to four statements which characterize how the counselor practices that quality in their professional helping relationships with clients. Research each term as it relates to Carl Rogers' people/client-centered therapy.

Congruence/Genuineness	Unconditional Positive Regard	Empathic Understanding

Part 2

In small groups, work through each quality, discussing each person's statements. Using chart paper or poster paper, develop a master list for each quality, blending, selecting, and validating the best statements. Include four to five statements for each quality.

Name ____________________ Date ____________ Class ____________

Lesson 14.2 Activity C

Key Terms Review

Review the lesson's key terms by matching the term with the example.

1. _____ Questions that cannot be answered with a static response, but instead require elaboration
2. _____ The ability to be fully present during the counseling session
3. _____ An attitude and behavior demonstrating esteem, honor, regard, concern, and other such positive qualities toward an individual, group, or entity
4. _____ A helping skill that uses questions to promote deeper understanding of the client's thoughts and feelings for both the counselor and the client
5. _____ The ability to be humble, characterized by a low focus on the self; an accurate sense of one's abilities, accomplishments, and worth; and an acknowledgment of one's limitations, imperfections, mistakes, and gaps in knowledge
6. _____ Involves paying attention to what the client is doing during treatment and when the counselor describes their personal response to the client
7. _____ Matching clients with providers according to cultural backgrounds
8. _____ The ability to not talk to allow the client time to think, feel, or form their response
9. _____ The counselor's ability to summarize or paraphrase back to the client their understanding of what the client has communicated
10. _____ A counselor's ability to effectively work with clients from different and/or specific cultures
11. _____ When you not only hear what someone is saying, but also make yourself receptive and aware of their thoughts and feelings
12. _____ Questions that can be answered with "yes" or "no"

A. active listening
B. attending
C. client-counselor match
D. closed questions
E. cultural competency
F. humility
G. immediacy
H. open-ended questions
I. questioning
J. reflecting
K. respect
L. silence

Name ______________________ Date ______________ Class ____________

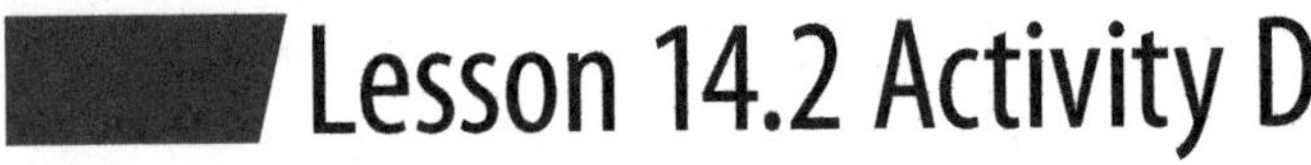

Lesson 14.2 Activity D

Helping Skill Skits

Working in pairs, you will develop two short skits that portray a snippet of a coaching or counseling session. Both skits will focus on portraying three of the helping skills listed below. Skit 1 will portray a coaching or counseling session without the three skills, while skit 2 will portray them being used in the same session.

Indicate the three skills you and your partner selected. Note: Your teacher may ask you to switch one out to make sure all skills are covered by at least one pair.

Acceptance
Active Listening
Attending
Authenticity/Genuineness
Calmness
Consistency
Empathy
Encouragement
Humility
Immediacy
Questioning
Rapport
Reflecting
Respect
Responsiveness
Silence
Warmth

Write your script using the table below. Practice with your partner and prepare to perform your two skits for the class.

Skit 1 (Ineffective Helping Skills)	Skit 2 (Effective Helping Skills)

Name ______________________ Date ____________ Class ____________

Lesson 14.2 Activity E

Practicing Helping Skills

Part 1: Naming Emotions

Read each situation and imagine what emotions the situation would trigger for you. Write down the emotions you imagine you would feel. Since people often mislabel emotions, consider referencing the glossary of your textbook, or search online for a feelings wheel. While there are no right or wrong answers for this activity, the more specific and precise you can be about emotions, the better prepared you will be for a career in counseling and mental health services.

1. You find out on social media that your best friend is now in a relationship with the person you both have been interested in for the last couple weeks.

____

____

2. You find out that your boss at work has scheduled you to work a shift that you had requested off so you could spend time with an extended family member. You really like this family member, who is stopping through for a night on their vacation.

____

____

3. You've been working really hard at practice and your coach has even commented on how improved you are. But on game night, she pulls you aside to tell you that while your work has not gone unnoticed, tonight's game is just too important to risk it and she'll be benching you most of the game.

____

____

4. You meet someone at a party who asks for your number and promises to call you the next day, but they don't.

____

____

5. A friend invites you out for dinner at your favorite restaurant and insists on paying the bill.

____

____

6. You're leaving a concert in a city you don't know very well, your friend's car won't start, and you both grab your cell phones only to discover they are both at less than 5% battery.

____

____

(Continued)

Part 2: Questioning

Next, for each comment that may be said by a client in session, write one open-ended question and one closed question you could ask as their counselor.

Client Session Scenario	Closed Question	Open-Ended Question
I've tried to talk to my husband several times about how annoying it is that he spends all weekend playing golf and hanging out with his friends.		
I don't think I can stay in school; I've got too much responsibility at home, and my family needs me.		
I just don't know what to do next. There are too many options.		
I've had a lot of problems with my boss. He's so annoying.		
I could never ask someone out! That's just not going to happen.		

Part 3: Reflection

Finally, practice reflecting back to the client your interpretation of the content and feelings conveyed in the statements below, to confirm you have the correct interpretation. NOTE: Your reflection should give the client the opportunity to confirm or help correct your interpretation, such as "So what I'm hearing is...Is that correct?"

1. I don't understand why I have to get a job that pays more to afford insurance and rent. I don't care about anything. I don't want to go back to school—absolutely not! I just want to start a family and take care of my kids.

 ____

 ____

2. Practically everyone I know is married! And, let's be honest, a lot are not great people. But here I am, a pretty good person, single in my 30s and alone. What's wrong with me? Maybe I'm not meant to fall in love.

 ____

 ____

3. I can't believe my friend's husband yelled at me like that in front of everyone. He said I was a "horrible person." Am I a horrible person? It was so embarrassing. It felt unreal. I rode with them to the restaurant, but I just ordered an Uber home to get out of there as quickly as possible.

 ____

 ____

4. So...I guess I'm here because I've been feeling down for a while. I'm not as happy at work as I used to be, I hate my body, I don't like going home because I have these roommates that just make a mess of my house....And a couple weeks ago, I was diagnosed with HIV. I just lie in bed and cry. It's all just more than I can handle.

 ____

 ____

Name ______________________ Date ____________ Class ____________

Lesson 14.3 Activity F

Key Terms Review

Answer the following questions to review the lesson's key terms.

1. What are the ground rules and limits of the client-helper relationship?

   ____

2. What is the process of the client and counselor working collaboratively to create therapeutic goals?

   ____

3. What occurs when there is incompatibility between an individual's or group's interests and motivations?

   ____

4. What is the principle of professional ethics that requires providers of mental health care or medical care to limit the disclosure of a client's or patient's identity, their condition or treatment, and any data entrusted to professionals?

   ____

5. Physical, emotional, or mental exhaustion accompanied by lowered motivation, performance, and attitudes toward oneself and others is called what?

   ____

6. What is the practice of establishing, communicating, and negotiating boundaries based on a variety of factors?

   ____

7. What occurs when a counselor has a second, significantly different relationship with their client in addition to their client-counselor relationship?

   ____

8. The act of revealing personal or private information about oneself to other people is called what?

   ____

9. What occurs when a provider projects past emotional reactions onto the present situation?

   ____

Name ______________________________ Date ______________ Class ____________

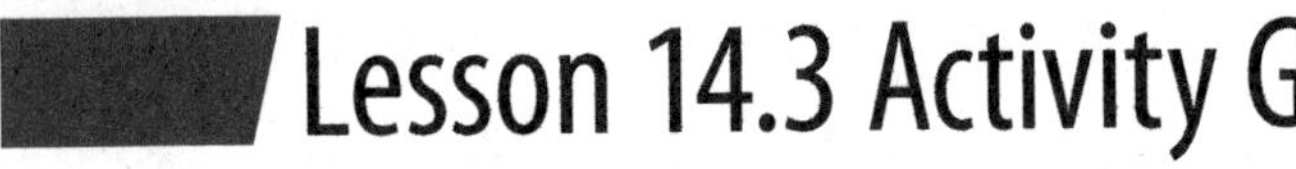

Lesson 14.3 Activity G

Observing Counseling Sessions and Taking Notes

There are many videos online of simulated counseling sessions. For this activity, either locate videos from reputable sources or use links provided by your teacher. During this activity, you will see several of the skills and techniques covered in this chapter while also practicing note taking.

Part 1

First, simply watch the video. As you watch, pause the video and jot down notes about the video: things you found interesting, things you wonder about, or things you observed that you have learned about. These notes are just for you about the video.

____

____

____

____

____

____

Part 2

Now that you finished with the video, imagine you are the counselor. The client has left the room, and you are going to record some notes from the session while it is still fresh in your mind. To do this, use the SOAP method outlined below. Note that session notes should be concise and only contain necessary information.

Parts of SOAP Method	Subjective	Objective	Assessment	Plan
Instructions	Briefly state what the client expressed as their experience and feelings from their perspective.	Include statements of fact or raw data that may support or contradict the subjective statements.	Provide a short statement of your interpretation of the client's situation. In the early days, these may start to point to a diagnosis, but they can also serve as progress notes.	Note any treatment provided in session, justification for that treatment, the client's response to treatment, next steps and appointments, follow-up items, "homework," and goals.
Session Notes				

Name ______________________ Date ____________ Class ____________

Lesson 14.3 Activity H

Helper Self-Care

Part 1

Review the survey statistics and answer the following questions about counselor self-care.

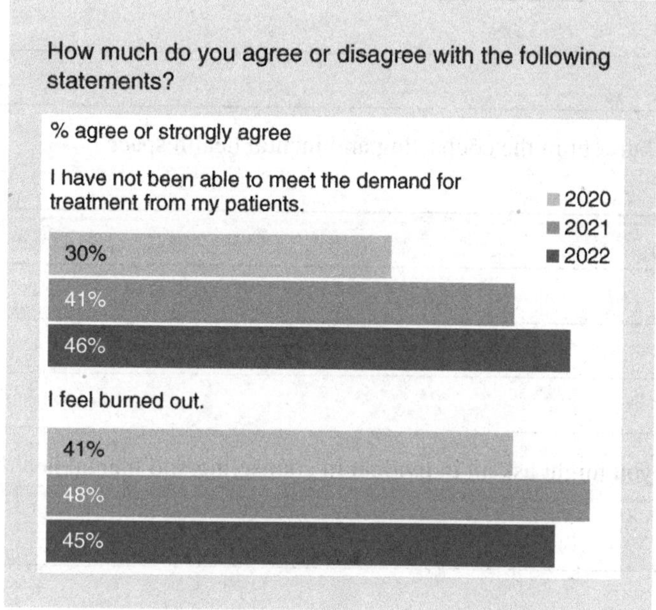

Goodheart-Willcox Publisher, data adapted from the American Psychological Association

1. What does the first bar graph indicate about the demand psychologists are facing?

____

2. What percentage of psychologists felt burnt out in 2021?

____

3. What percentage of psychologists felt burnt out in 2022?

____

4. What conclusions can you draw about psychologists' workloads by looking at both graphs?

____

____

____

(Continued)

Part 2

Answer the following reflection questions.

1. Why is it important for counselors to practice self-care?

2. What are some causes of burnout in the counseling and mental health space?

3. Write two questions that you might ask an individual in counseling and mental health to see if they are experiencing burnout.

4. Describe two forms of self-care you will practice when you enter a career in counseling and mental health and how it might help you prevent burnout in your career.

Name ______ Date ______ Class ______

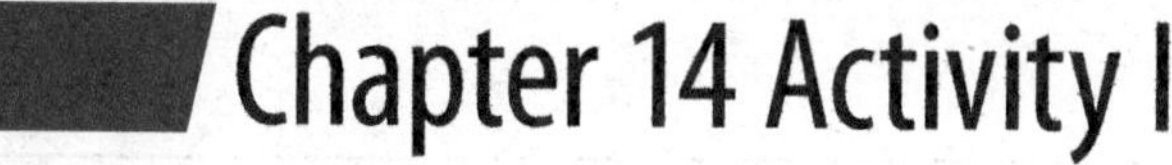

Chapter 14 Activity I

Chapter Review

Lesson 14.1 Professional Helping Relationships

Answer the following question.

1. What are the three phases of mental health treatment, in order of most rapid change to slowest change?

______

______

Mark each statement as E for effective counselor approaches or I for ineffective counselor approaches.

2. ______ Reduces the client to their diagnosis
3. ______ Sensitive to client attitudes and moods
4. ______ Seeks to understand the client's beliefs, values, meanings, and feelings
5. ______ Uses standard therapeutic goals focused on relieving the symptoms of a mental health disorder
6. ______ Actively and personally participating in the relationship
7. ______ Emphasizes past history

List characteristics and skills of helping relationships. The first letter of each is provided for you.

8. T ______
9. G ______
10. A ______
11. W ______
12. E ______

Lesson 14.2 Helping Skills

Answer the following questions.

1. Name the three stages in Clara E. Hill's model of helping.

______

2. What two contexts surround these stages in Hill's model?

______

Recall the S-O-L-E-R method for attending skills by filling in the blanks below.

3. Face the other person ______.

______

4. Adopt a(n) ______ posture.

______

(Continued)

5. _____ slightly toward the other person.

____

6. Maintain good _____ contact.

____

7. Stay _____.

____

Answer the following questions.

8. _____ Which coaching model builds rapport and trust, and involves deeper collaboration and analysis of intrapersonal factors?
   A. CLEAR B. GROW C. OSCAR D. SOLER

9. _____ Which coaching model is best used for a single coaching session or meeting, or to address a specific situation or challenge?
   A. CLEAR B. GROW C. OSCAR D. SOLER

Lesson 14.3 Managing Treatment

For each statement, indicate if the statement is True or False. If False, explain how to correct the statement to make it True.

1. If the client's expectations are unrealistic, helpers should clarify expectations at a later session.

____

2. If the counselor has strong negative countertransference reactions to the client, then they should refer the client to another helper.

____

3. Professional counselors manage confidentiality solely around the legal protections that exist for clients.

____

4. The counselor determines the focus of the session.

____

5. To maximize time during a session, counselors should initiate new topics within the last ten minutes.

____

6. One way to analyze and process therapeutic sessions is by taking notes after each session.

____

7. Notes on manifest content are the unspoken meanings in what the client said.

____

8. According to the APA, therapists should terminate when they feel they are no longer working productively.

____

Name ______________________ Date ______________ Class ______________

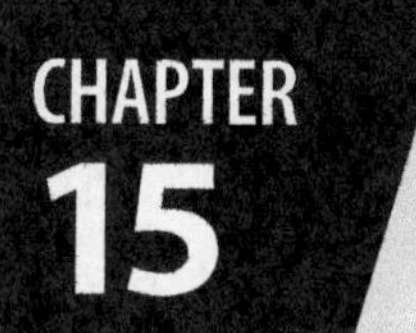

The Business of Counseling and Mental Health

Lesson 15.1 Activity A

Key Terms Review

Fill in the blanks of the following statements to review the lesson's key terms.

1. A contractual relationship in which an insurer agrees to pay all or some of the insured person's healthcare costs in exchange for a monthly or annual premium is called _____.

   ____

2. _____ refers to an individual's ability to receive mental health services and treatment.

   ____

3. The _____ describes the procedures, actions, and processes that a worker is permitted to undertake in keeping with the terms of their professional license.

   ____

4. _____ are the privately owned components within the mental health system that either directly provide or provide access to mental health services and treatment.

   ____

5. All the activities and efforts geared toward building a population that meets the needs of the economy, employers, and the labor market is called _____.

   ____

6. The _____ includes the separate services, activities, and policies in place to address mental health issues at the individual, family, and community levels.

   ____

7. A(n) _____ is a set of standards adopted by organizations to assist their members in understanding the difference between right and wrong, and knowing how to apply that understanding to their decisions.

   ____

8. _____ means having federal, state, or local government agencies or departments work together to address specific mental health issues.

   ____

9. A(n) _____ is an identification of strengths, weaknesses, opportunities, and threats in the mental health system.

   ____

10. _____ are the government-run components within the mental health system that either directly provide or provide access to mental health services and treatment.

   ____

Name ______________________ Date ______________ Class ____________

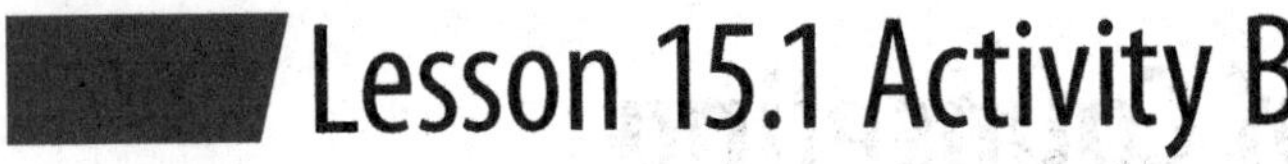

Lesson 15.1 Activity B

SWOT Analysis

Working in small groups, conduct a SWOT analysis of your local mental health system. This may involve online research, resource mapping, interviewing professionals, and conducting a survey.

Internal

Strengths	Weaknesses

External

Opportunities	Threats

Name ____________________ Date ____________ Class ____________

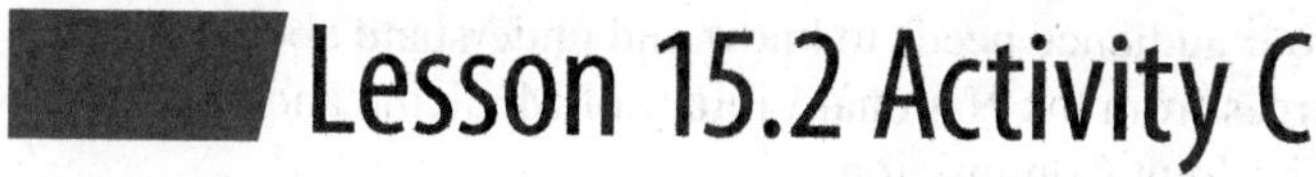

Lesson 15.2 Activity C

Patient Safety and Risk Management in Mental Health

For this activity, you will dive deeper into patient safety and risk management in mental health, while also applying concepts about communicating information. Your teacher will assign you one of the three situations below. Assuming the role provided, develop a presentation for the audience, format, and topic indicated.

Component	Situation #1	Situation #2	Situation #3
Role	Clinical Supervisor	Psychiatric Facility Administrator	Dept. of Health & Human Services Licensure & Training Consultant
Audience	Mental Health Counselors	All Facility Staff	Facility Administrators
Format	New mental health counselor training	Safety protocols refresher presentation	Initial certification class for behavioral health facility administrators
Topic	Medical Errors in Psychiatric Care	Adverse Events in Patients Receiving Mental Healthcare	Safety Practices and Implementation Strategies

Part 1: Research

Complete the outline below to capture your research and prepare your presentation.

1. What do you know about your role? Research your role and capture a few bullet points that describe the responsibilities of that role.

____

____

____

____

____

____

____

____

2. Reflecting on your assigned role, capture a few bullet points that will help you frame your messages for your audiences. What should be the objectives of your presentation? What is their experience or technical knowledge of the topic? What depth of knowledge do they need? What kind of words may you need to define?

____

____

____

____

____

____

____

____

(Continued)

3. Research your topic and summarize the main points your audience needs to know and understand about your topic. As a starting place for your research, visit resources from the National Library of Medicine and behavioral health and human services goals and standards from The Joint Commission.

4. What type of activity can you incorporate into your presentation to engage the audience and check to see if they are understanding?

Part 2

Develop and deliver your presentation using the presentation technology and resources as provided and directed by your teacher.

Name ______________________ Date ______________ Class ______________

Lesson 15.2 Activity D

Key Terms Review

Review the lesson's key terms by matching the term with the example.

1. _____ A client's voluntary agreement to participate in a procedure after understanding the procedure, its possible risks and benefits, and available alternatives
2. _____ A safety mindset in which all human bodily fluids are presumed to carry infectious disease
3. _____ Type of insurance that covers professional errors and financial loss from negligence
4. _____ A federal law that establishes national standards to protect individuals' medical records and other individually identifiable health information
5. _____ A process that involves assessing, planning, coordinating, monitoring, and evaluating, all of which are tailored to the individual client's needs
6. _____ The process of identifying, analyzing, and accepting or mitigating possible harm to a person or operation
7. _____ The health information protected by HIPAA
8. _____ A failure to fulfill a duty or to provide some response, action, or level of care that is appropriate or reasonable to expect
9. _____ Research method that involves interpreting words, symbols, or observations to understand subjective phenomena and grouping data to find consistent patterns or themes
10. _____ Type of insurance that mitigates the risk of financial losses associated with injury or damage to personal property
11. _____ The process of converting readable plaintext into unreadable ciphertext that can be converted back to plaintext only by authorized individuals
12. _____ A mental health team made up of a variety of professional staff
13. _____ Professional misconduct or negligent behavior on the part of a practitioner that may lead to legal action
14. _____ Research method that collects numerical data and uses objective measurements and statistical analysis
15. _____ A defendant's legal responsibility to pay monetary damages for injury or other harm that a court deems they have caused the plaintiff

A. case management
B. data encryption
C. general public liability insurance
D. Health Insurance Portability and Accountability Act (HIPAA)
E. informed consent
F. liability
G. malpractice
H. multidisciplinary team (MDT)
I. negligence
J. protected health information (PHI)
K. professional indemnity insurance
L. qualitative research
M. quantitative research
N. risk management
O. universal precautions

Name ______________________________ Date ______________ Class __________

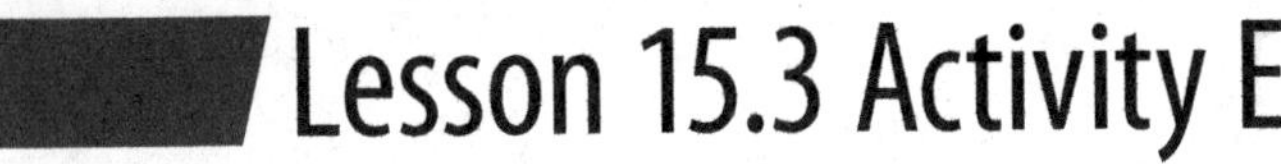

Lesson 15.3 Activity E

Key Terms Review

Part 1

Answer the following questions to review the lesson's key terms.

1. What is a streamlined version of a business plan that can be used to sketch out and communicate the entrepreneurial venture?

 ____

2. What is the money set aside to earn revenue to fund charitable activities?

 ____

3. What is the primary legal document of the organization that establishes its name, mission, and initial board members?

 ____

4. A person who starts a business, organization, or venture for the greater social good and not just the pursuit of profits is called what?

 ____

5. What are legal entities that are organized and operated to provide a collective or social benefit rather than to generate a profit for owners?

 ____

6. What is the secondary legal document of the organization that serves as a set of rules for how the organization will run?

 ____

Part 2

Label the parts of the life cycle of a nonprofit organization in order from 1 to 6.

1. _____ Maturity
2. _____ Growth
3. _____ Idea
4. _____ Decline
5. _____ Start-up
6. _____ Crisis

Name ______________________ Date ____________ Class ____________

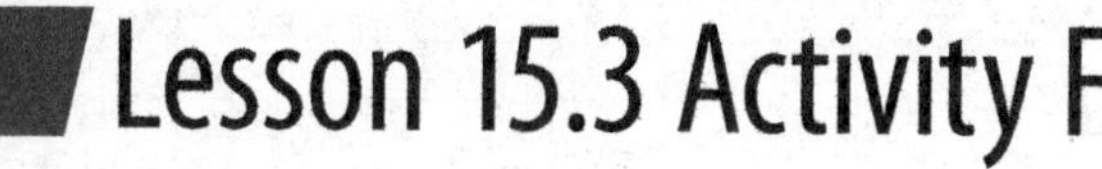

Lesson 15.3 Activity F

Entrepreneur Self-Assessment

For each of the traits of an entrepreneur below, rank yourself on a scale of 1 to 10. Then, complete the reflection questions.

Trait	Scale
Adaptivity	
Comfort with failure	
Confidence	
Curiosity	
Decisiveness	
Determination	
Ethics and integrity	
Innovative thinking	
Leadership	
Long-term focus	
Persistence	
Problem-solving	
Risk tolerance	
Self-awareness	
Self-motivation	
Willingness to experiment	

1. How can you imagine using entrepreneurial skills in a career in counseling, mental health, or human services?

2. What are two traits you might want to work on developing? How could you go about developing them?

3. Why do you think these two skills are important for leading human services teams and organizations?

Name ______________________ Date ____________ Class ____________

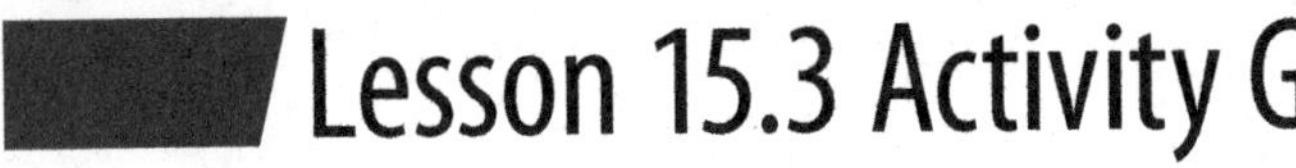

Lesson 15.3 Activity G

Exploring Nonprofit Organizations

Choose a nonprofit organization to research.

Part 1: Research a Nonprofit Organization

Prompt	Response
Nonprofit Name	
Website	
Mission	
Vision	
Values or Purpose	
Social Media Accounts	
Who does the organization serve?	
What type of work does the organization participate in?	
What are some examples of staff positions that the organization has? What is the leadership structure?	

Part 2: Summary

1. What did you find most interesting about the nonprofit you researched?

____

____

____

2. Reviewing your nonprofit, can you tell what part of the nonprofit life cycle they are currently experiencing?

____

____

3. Would you be interested in working for this nonprofit in the future? Why or why not?

____

____

____

____

Name ______________________ Date ____________ Class ____________

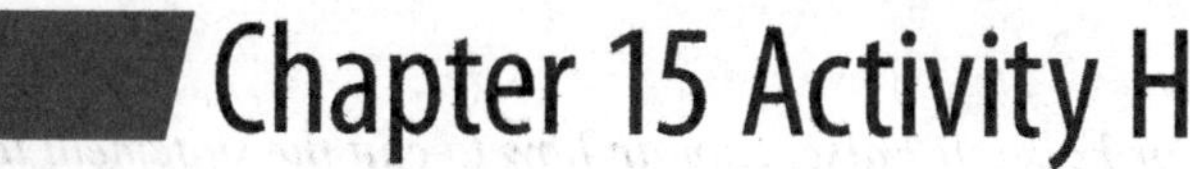

Chapter 15 Activity H

Chapter Review

Lesson 15.1 Mental Health System

Classify each of the mental health system components into their appropriate category.

American Psychological Association (APA)	**Medicare, Medicaid, and TRICARE**	**State psychiatric hospitals**
Colleges and universities	**Mental health laws**	**Substance Abuse and Mental Health Services Administration (SAMHSA)**
Elementary and secondary schools	**National Institute of Mental Health (NIMH)**	**US Department of Health and Human Services (HHS)**
Health insurance companies	**Nonprofit mental health providers**	**Veterans Affairs (VA) clinics**
Local health departments	**Small mental health practices**	

Private Service Providers	Public Service Providers	Regulatory Agencies, Policies, and Advocacy	Education, Research, and Workforce Development

Answer the following questions.

1. _____ What component in the mental health system provides funding through a contractual relationship to help people pay for mental health services?
   A. FDA
   B. Health insurance
   C. State licensing boards
   D. State developmental centers

2. _____ Which of the following is *not* a barrier to accessing mental health services?
   A. Paying for services
   B. Transportation to/from services
   C. Stigma around mental health treatment
   D. Providing additional resources to support special populations

3. _____ What are rules created by government human services departments that impact the mental health system?
   A. Administrative codes
   B. Administrative hearings
   C. Bills
   D. Laws

4. _____ Which mental health system component is focused on directing the attention of policymakers, clinicians, and the public to mental health issues and concerns?
   A. Advocacy organizations and activities
   B. Education and research
   C. Professional associations
   D. Workforce development

5. _____ Which mental health system component supports having well-trained human services assistants, mental health nurses, mental health counselors, psychiatrists, and neuropsychologists?
   A. Advocacy organizations and activities
   B. Education and research
   C. Professional associations
   D. Workforce development

(Continued)

Lesson 15.2 Management

For each statement below, indicate if the statement is True or False. If False, explain how to edit the statement to make it True.

1. Good management in counseling and mental health services can result in improved client outcomes.

   ____

2. The Food and Drug Administration (FDA) provides a training and certification program that promotes general workplace safety and health.

   ____

3. Clinicians should take care to inform clients and ensure they fully understand and consent to treatment and services.

   ____

4. The final two stages of case management are implementing and ongoing follow-up.

   ____

5. Information management is the appropriate and optimized capture, storage, retrieval, and use of information.

   ____

6. Student health information held by a school generally is subject to HIPAA.

   ____

7. Virtual reality can help protect employee data and client-protected health information.

   ____

Lesson 15.3 Marketing and Social Entrepreneurship

Answer the following questions.

1. List and explain the four Ps of marketing mental health services:

   ____

   ____

   ____

   ____

   ____

2. What are the 6 Ps of social entrepreneurship?

   ____

   ____

3. What tool can social entrepreneurs use to plan their venture and solicit startup funding from donors?

   ____

4. What are the six stages within the life cycle of nonprofit organizations?

   ____

   ____

5. Who hires and evaluates the executive director or chief executive officer of a nonprofit organization?

   ____

Name ______ Date ______ Class ______

CHAPTER 16

Your Career Development

Lesson 16.1 Activity A

Key Terms Review

Fill in the blanks in the following statements to review the lesson's key terms.

1. ______ is an educational experience that enhances classroom learning by connecting it to the workplace.

______

2. A(n) ______ is an authorization, typically from a state government or board, for a person to provide certain services within that state.

______

3. ______ is where a person observes a professional perform their work, typically for one to two days.

______

4. A confidential process where trained students act as neutral mediators to help their peers resolve conflicts is called ______.

______

5. ______ is a foundational project management tool to use when designing interventions that address personal, work, and societal issues.

______

6. A(n) ______ is a statistical projection of job growth and job openings that, if it holds true, can serve as an indicator of the demand for certain occupations.

______

7. ______ is a period of specialized medical training in a hospital.

______

8. ______ is a national career and technical student organization for students exploring and preparing for careers that support individuals, families, and communities.

______

9. A(n) ______ is when a student begins practicing counseling theories in real-world situations under supervision.

______

10. ______ focus on the growth and well-being of people and the communities to which they belong.

______

Name ____________________ Date ____________ Class ____________

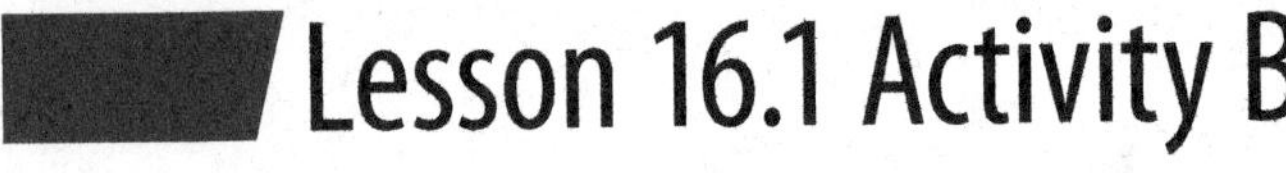

Lesson 16.1 Activity B

Professional Association Recruitment Campaign

Part 1

Select one of the professional associations from Figure 16.6 that you want to learn more about, or that is related to a career you are interested in pursuing or learning more about. Research that professional association and develop a brand asset that would be used to recruit members. You can select the brand asset from the choice board below.

10 Social media posts and images	1 2-minute video	2 Webpages
1 10-minute podcast mini-episode (interview-format)	1 500-800 word article/story/blog	2 Media-rich email flier
1 Large poster	1 3-minute parody song (writing your own lyrics to an existing song)	3 Infographics

Part 2

Working in small groups, collaborate with your peers to create a communications plan for a month-long membership recruitment campaign for one of these professional associations. What brand assets are needed? When should they be deployed? What is the theme? What are the key messages?

Name ______________________ Date ______________ Class ____________

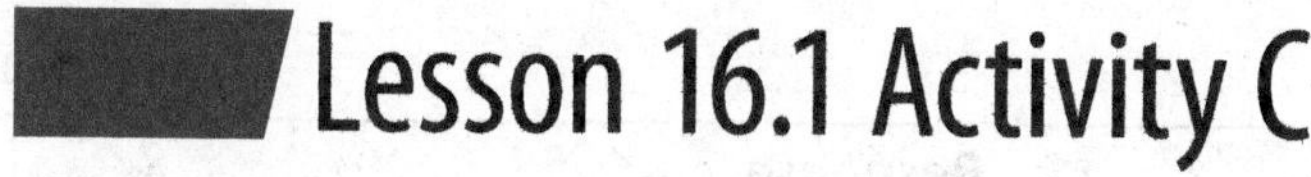

Lesson 16.1 Activity C

Peer Mediation Activity

For this activity, two pairs of students will work together, forming a team of four. Each pair will collaborate to create a fake conflict to practice peer mediation. During the first round, one pair will play the role of two students in conflict, and the other pair will serve as peer mediators. During the second round, the pairs will swap roles.

Round 1

Prompt	Response
Notes about Conflict/ Situation/Context	
Outcomes/Resolution	
Things Mediator Did Well (Strategies, Skills, Techniques)	
Mediator Opportunities for Improvement	

Round 2

Prompt	Response
Notes about Conflict/ Situation/Context	
Outcomes/Resolution	
Things Mediator Did Well (Strategies, Skills, Techniques)	
Mediator Opportunities for Improvement	

(Continued)

Peer Mediation Contract

Prompt	Response
Date	
Disputants' commitment	1. I am willing to try to solve my problem through mediation. 2. Only one person talks at a time. 3. There should be no name-calling or put-downs. 4. We both need to tell the truth. 5. There is to be no physical fighting, yelling, or throwing things. 6. Everything of a personal nature must be kept confidential. 7. If something I say would harm me, each other, or anyone else, it will be reported to an administrator.
Disputant #1 name and grade	
Disputant #1 signature	
Disputant #2 name and grade	
Disputant #2 signature	
Peer mediators' commitment	1. We will not take sides. 2. We will not judge or try to punish you. We will not tell you how to solve this conflict. 3. We will help you solve your conflict. 4. We will help you put your agreement in writing. 5. We will keep confidential what you tell us today (unless it involves drugs, weapons, or threat of harm to yourself or others). 6. We will give a copy of your agreement to our program coordinator.
Peer Mediator #1 signature	
Peer Mediator #2 signature	

Peer Mediation Outline

PROBLEM: The two disputants listed above came to Peer Mediation for help with the following problem:

____

____

____

____

SOLUTION: The two disputants agreed to the following options:

1. ____
2. ____
3. ____
4. ____
5. ____

AGREEMENT: The two disputants agreed that they will do the following should this happen again:

____

____

____

Name ______________________________ Date ______________ Class ______________

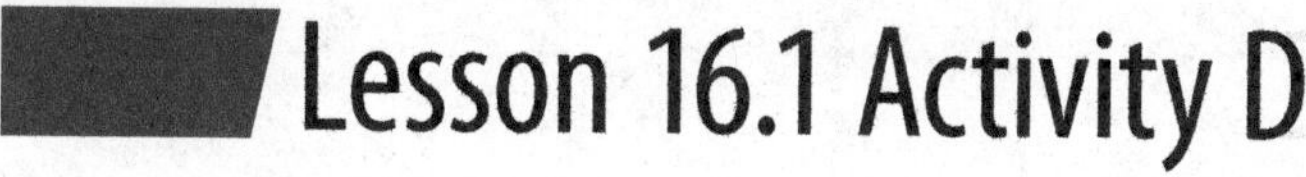

Lesson 16.1 Activity D

Informational Interview

Conduct an interview with a professional in the field of counseling and mental health services. Create questions to ask the professional to learn more about the experience.

Part 1

Ask these standard questions of the person being interviewed (the interviewee).

Prompt	Response
Name of Interviewee	
Business or Organization	
Title of Interviewee	
Describe the activities associated with the position.	
What type of education or training was required for the position?	
What is a typical workday in your position?	

Part 2

Write five additional questions you would like answered by the interviewee. Write the questions and answers below.

Prompt	Question	Response
Question 1		
Question 2		
Question 3		
Question 4		
Question 5		

Name ________________ Date ________ Class ________

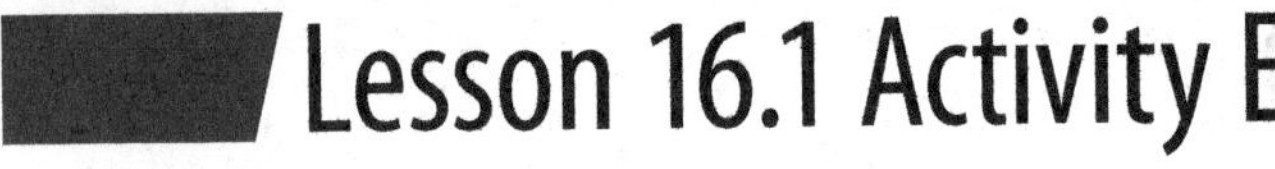

Lesson 16.1 Activity E

Job Shadowing

Select a job shadowing experience to complete this activity. Spend a day with a professional and complete this activity as part of it.

Prompt	Response
Name of Person You Are Shadowing	
Business or Organization	
Title of Person You Are Shadowing	
Describe the activities associated with the position.	
What type of education or training was required for the position?	
What other skills or duties did you notice the person needed for the position?	
Describe the work environment you visited.	
Write three qualities that you think would be helpful in a position like this.	
Would this be a position you would be interested in doing? Why or why not?	
Is there anything else you would like to share about your experience?	

Name ______________________ Date ____________ Class ____________

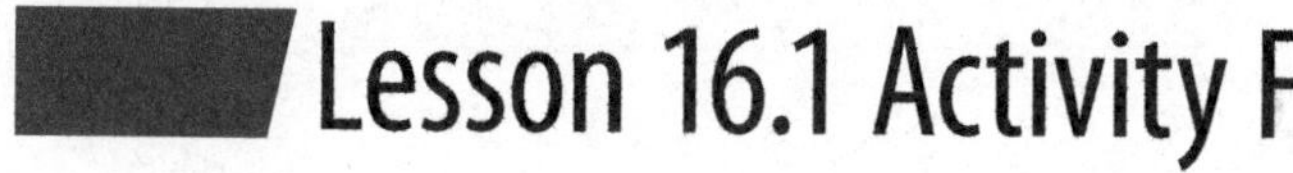

Lesson 16.1 Activity F

FCCLA Planning Process Activity

Use the FCCLA Planning Process to develop a project that promotes mental health within your school or community.

Planning Process Step		Description of This Step in Your Project
	Identify concerns.	
	Set a goal.	
	Form a plan (who, what, when, where, how, cost, resources, and evaluation).	
	Act.	
	Follow up.	

Name ______________________ Date ____________ Class ____________

Lesson 16.2 Activity G

Key Terms Review

Review the lesson's key terms by matching the term with the example.

1. _____ The trail of data you leave behind when using the internet, including traceable digital activities, actions, contributions, and communications
2. _____ A fellow worker in the same profession or organization, who often holds a similar rank or status
3. _____ The intentional process of defining and promoting one's unique mix of professional values, traits, skills, experiences, and credentials
4. _____ Event with employers looking to fill vacancies now
5. _____ Includes the jobs that are filled before they are posted or made public
6. _____ The media that help communicate and promote the brand to others
7. _____ The process of interacting with people who are connected to career fields, industries, and employers that interest you
8. _____ A brief account of a person's education, qualifications, and previous experience
9. _____ Event designed to increase your awareness of occupations, industries, and employers

A. brand assets
B. career fair
C. colleague
D. digital footprint
E. hidden job market
F. job fair
G. networking
H. personal branding
I. résumé

Name ______________________ Date ____________ Class ____________

Lesson 16.2 Activity H

Practice Writing BAQQR Bullet Statements

Remember that BAQQR statements are bullets that start with action verbs (like "Evaluated," "Directed," "Managed," "Coordinated," "Supervised," or "Created"), include the task that was completed with enough important context (who, what, when, where, and how), incorporate any numbers that show significance (like how long you worked in a certain position), and any results that were gained or accomplished from the task. Practice writing BAQQR bullet statements for your own career and academic accomplishments.

- ______________________
- ______________________
- ______________________
- ______________________
- ______________________
- ______________________
- ______________________
- ______________________
- ______________________
- ______________________

Name ______________________ Date ______________ Class ____________

Lesson 16.2 Activity I

Job and Career Fair Preparation

Answer the following question.

1. Compare and contrast job fairs and career fairs.

____

____

____

Write three questions you might ask potential employers at a job fair about their specific positions.

2. ____

____

3. ____

____

4. ____

____

Write five questions you would ask potential employers at a career fair to find out more about the careers in their industry.

5. ____

____

6. ____

____

7. ____

____

8. ____

____

9. ____

____

Finally, answer the following question.

10. Which event would be more useful for you to attend at this stage in your career development? Why?

____

____

____

Name ____________________ Date ____________ Class ____________

Chapter 16 Activity J

Chapter Review

Lesson 16.1 Career Leadership and Development

Answer the following questions.

1. What are the seven components of a career development plan?

____

____

____

____

____

2. List four important practices for peer mediators.

____

____

____

____

3. _____ Who would be *most likely* to complete a residency as part of their professional preparation?
   A. Marriage and family therapist
   B. Psychiatrist
   C. Psychologist
   D. Social worker

4. _____ Renewing a license involves documentation of professional development, also referred to as _____.
   A. career advancement
   B. continuing education
   C. education and training
   D. training and development

5. _____ Which is *not* a method of professional development?
   A. Attending conferences
   B. Reading professional journals
   C. Obtaining specialized certifications
   D. Protecting client confidentiality

6. _____ Which organization allows secondary students to begin developing career and leadership skills they can apply to a career in counseling and mental health services?
   A. APA
   B. ICF
   C. FCCLA
   D. NCDA

7. _____ Which should you *not* do when experiencing failure?
   A. Ask for feedback from people you trust.
   B. Reflect on what you may try differently in the future.
   C. Celebrate and honor the fact you had the courage to try.
   D. Focus on the criticism of those who have avoided vulnerability.

8. _____ Which is a characteristic of a servant leader?
   A. Measures success through accomplishment alone
   B. Seeks to obtain a rank, degree, or accolade
   C. Understands it is not about them
   D. Uses power and control

9. _____ When using the FCCLA Planning Process, what should you do *before* setting a goal?
   A. Act.
   B. Follow up.
   C. Form a plan.
   D. Identify concerns.

(Continued)

10. _____ When using the FCCLA Planning Process, what should you do *after* setting a goal?
A. Act.
B. Follow up.
C. Form a plan.
D. Identify concerns.

Lesson 16.2 Marketing Yourself

For each statement, indicate if it is True or False. If False, indicate how to correct the statement to make it True.

1. Studies suggest that job boards are the most successful job search strategy, making it an essential career development skill that you can begin practicing now.

____

2. A brief description of who you are and what you want to accomplish in your career is referred to as a "pitch" or "elevator speech."

____

3. When networking, you never know who may be able to help you, so you should pursue a connection with someone who seems overly negative or pessimistic or like they are not interested in helping and supporting your career goals.

____

4. Your personal brand should *not* reflect your character, values, and personality.

____

5. Remember the adage, "Dance like nobody's watching, but text, email, and post like it will be read in court one day."

____

6. Many employers are increasingly using digital screening software and artificial intelligence (AI) to narrow the pool of résumés before they are even reviewed by a person.

____

Answer the following questions.

7. _____ When applying the STAR Method to responding to interview questions, the "A" represents _____.
A. accomplishments achieved
B. adaptation to situation
C. access to information
D. actions taken

8. _____ When applying the STAR Method to responding to interview questions, the "R" represents _____.
A. reframe positively
B. results or outcome
C. reassess interventions
D. react to concerns

9. _____ Which is something a person should *not* do when preparing for a job interview?
A. Practice with friends and family prior to the interview.
B. Preplan some questions to ask the interviewer.
C. Allow plenty of time to arrive and walk in 30 minutes early.
D. Project confidence by making eye contact with interviewers, smiling, talking slowly and calmly, and avoiding fidgeting.

10. _____ Which would *least likely* be asked in a counseling and mental health services job interview?
A. "What religion do you practice?"
B. "How do you maintain your mental health?"
C. "How do you approach creating a treatment plan?"
D. "How do you approach situations where the client is struggling to open up to you?"